DELMAR

T0200658

# Mini Guide

## to Geriatric Drugs

**George R. Spratto, PhD**

Dean Emeritus and Professor

School of Pharmacy

West Virginia University

Morgantown, West Virginia

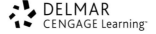

DELMAR

CENGAGE Learning™

## NOTICE TO THE READER

The monographs in *Delmar's Mini Guide to Geriatric Drugs* is the work of distinguished author George R. Spratto, PhD, Dean Emeritus and Professor of Pharmacology of the School of Pharmacy at West Virginia University, Morgantown, West Virginia.

The publisher and the author do not warrant or guarantee any of the products described herein or perform any independent analysis in connection with any of the product information contained herein. The publisher and the author do not assume and expressly disclaim any obligation to obtain and include information other than that provided by the manufacturer.

The reader is expressly warned to consider and adopt all safety precautions that might be indicated by the activities described herein and to avoid all potential hazards. By following the instructions contained herein, the reader willingly assumes all risks in connection with such instructions.

The publisher and the author make no representations or warranties of any kind, including but not limited to the warranties of fitness for a particular purpose or merchantability nor are any such representations implied with respect to the material set forth herein, and the publisher and the author take no responsibility with respect to such material. The publisher and the author shall not be liable for any special, consequential, or exemplary damages resulting, in whole or in part, from the reader's use of, or reliance upon, this material.

The author and publisher have made a conscientious effort to ensure that the drug information and recommended dosages in this book and companion web site are accurate and in accord with accepted standards at the time of publication. However, pharmacology and therapeutics are rapidly changing sciences, so readers are advised, before administering any drug, to check the package insert provided by the manufacturer for the recommended dose, for any contraindications for administration, and for any added warnings and precautions. This recommendation is especially important for new, infrequently used, or highly toxic drugs.

# TABLE OF CONTENTS

# PREFACE

*Delmar's Mini Guide to Geriatric Drugs* consists of approximately 100 drugs that may be prescribed or used in geriatric clients. The cards are intended to be a quick reference source for important information about the drug.

## USING THE DRUG CARDS

The following components are described in the order in which they appear on the cards. Please note that the information presented for each drug is not comprehensive; the reader should consult other sources, such as *Delmar 2010 Edition Nurse's Drug Handbook*™, for more complete information.

- **Drug Name:** The generic drug name is the first item in the name block (in color at the beginning of each monograph).
- **Phonetic Pronunciation:** All generic drug names include phonetic pronunciation.
- **Trade Name:** Trade names are identified as OTC (over-the-counter, no prescription required) or Rx (prescription).
- ■ **Black Box Warning:** The black box icon indicates that the FDA has issued a boxed warning about potentially dangerous or life-threatening side effects. The actual black box warning is found in the accompanying online companion (OLC), available at http://www.delmarlearning.com/companions.
- **Pregnancy Category:** The FDA pregnancy category (A, B, C, D, or X) assigned to the drug is indicated.
- **Controlled Substance:** If the drug is controlled by the U.S. Federal Controlled Substances Act, the schedule in which the drug is placed (C-II, C-III, C-IV, or C-V) follows the trade name listing.
- **Classification:** The type of drug or the drug class under which the drug is listed is defined.
- **Uses:** Approved therapeutic uses for the drug in the geriatric population are included. Note that the drug may be used for the same or other purposes in other populations of clients.
- **Action/Kinetics:** The action portion describes the proposed mechanism(s) by which a drug achieves its therapeutic effect. Not all mechanisms of action are known, and some are self-evident, as when a hormone is administered as a replacement. The kinetics portion lists critical information, if known, about the rate of drug absorption (including, when known, the percent bioavailable), distribution, time for peak plasma levels or peak effect, minimum effective serum or plasma levels, biological half-life, duration of action, metabolism, and ex-

cretion route(s). Metabolism and excretion may be important for clients with systemic liver disease, kidney disease, or both.

The half-life (t ½—the time required for one-half the drug to be excreted or removed from the blood, serum, or plasma) is important in determining how often a drug is to be administered and how long the client is to be assessed for side effects. Therapeutic levels indicate the desired concentration, in serum or plasma, for the drug to exert its beneficial effect and are helpful in predicting the onset of side effects or lack of drug effect.

- **Side Effects:** Listed are the most common undesired or bothersome effects the client may experience while taking a particular drug. In addition, potentially life-threatening side effects are displayed in red italics. Note that the side effects presented are not comprehensive for that particular drug.

- **Dosage:** The dosage form/route of administration and disease state (both in color) for use in the geriatric client are given followed by the dosage for the geriatric client. For ease of reading, shading separates dosages for various uses.

The listed dosage is to be considered as a general guideline; the exact amount of the drug to be given is determined by the provider. However, one should question orders when dosages differ markedly from the accepted norm. Note that the same or other dosage forms, routes of administration, uses, and dosages may be appropriate for other groups of clients. Appropriate sources should be consulted for this information.

- **Need to Know:** This numbered list provides information on important contraindications, special concerns, drug interactions, and nursing considerations (including administration and client information) for the geriatric client. This list is not intended to be complete; the reader must consult more comprehensive resources for this information.

# ACKNOWLEDGMENTS

I would like to extend my thanks and appreciation to the Delmar Cengage Learning team who works so diligently to ensure that the manuscript process flows smoothly and keeps the schedule moving. Team members include Matthew Kane, Director of Learning Solutions; Maureen Rosener, Senior Acquisitions Editor; Beth Williams, Senior Product Manager; Stacey Lamodi, Senior Content Project Manager; Jack Pendleton, Senior Art Director; Mary Colleen Liburdi, Senior Technology Product Manager; and Erin Zeggert, Technology Project Manager.

I also extend greatest appreciation and love to my wife, Lynne, as well as my son Chris and his family (daughter-in-law Mary Alice and grandchildren Patrick Santopietro and Victoria Santopietro) and my son Gregg and his family (daughter-in-law Kim and grandchildren Alexandra and Dominic)—all of whom make the work of this project worthwhile by their unfailing support and encouragement.

**George Spratto**

**CLASSIFICATION(S):** Bone growth regulator, bisphosphonate

**USES: Daily dosing:** (1) Prevent osteoporosis in women who are at risk of developing osteoporosis and to maintain bone mass and reduce the risk of future fracture. (2) Treat osteoporosis in postmenopausal women to increase bone mass and reduce the incidence of fractures, including those of the hip and spine. (3) Increase bone density in men with osteoporosis. (4) Glucocorticoid-induced osteoporosis in men and women receiving daily dosage equivalent to 7.5 mg or greater of prednisone and who have low bone mineral density. Used with adequate amounts of calcium and Vitamin D. **Weekly dosing:** Treatment or prevention of postmenopausal osteoporosis in women or osteoporosis in men.

**ACTION/KINETICS:** Binds to bone hydroxyapatite and inhibits osteoclast activity, thereby preventing bone resorption. Appears to reduce fracture risk and reverse the progression of osteoporosis. Well absorbed orally and initially distributed to soft tissues, but then quickly redistributed to bone. Not metabolized; excreted through the urine. **t½, terminal:** Believed to be more than 10 years, due to slow release from the skeleton.

**SIDE EFFECTS:** Abdominal pain, dyspepsia, nausea, constipation, diarrhea.

---

**DOSAGE: Oral Solution; Tablets**

*Prevention of osteoporosis in postmenopausal women.*
   **Adults:** One 35-mg tablet once weekly or one 5-mg tablet once daily.

*Treatment of osteoporosis in postmenopausal women.*
   **Adults:** One 70-mg tablet once weekly, one 10-mg tablet once daily, or 1 bottle of 70 mg oral solution once weekly.

*Osteoporosis in men.*
   **Adults:** One 70-mg tablet once weekly, one 10-mg tablet once daily, or 1 bottle of 70 mg oral solution once weekly.

*Glucocorticoid-induced osteoporosis.*
   **Adults:** One 5-mg tablet once daily for men and women. For postmenopausal women not receiving estrogen, the recommended dose is one 10-mg tablet daily. Also give clients adequate amounts of calcium and vitamin D.

## NEED TO KNOW

1. Use with caution in those with upper GI problems, such as dysphagia, symptomatic esophageal diseases, gastritis, duodenitis, or ulcers.
2. To facilitate stomach delivery and reduce esophagus irritation, do not lie down for at least 30 min following administration.
3. Due to possible interference with absorption, at least 30 min should elapse before taking antacids or calcium supplements.
4. No dosage adjustment needed for the elderly.
5. Take as prescribed. Benefit seen only when each tablet is taken with 6–8 oz of plain water first thing in the morning at least 30 min before the first food, beverage, or medication of the day. Remain upright. Waiting more than 30 min will improve absorption. Taking with juice or coffee will markedly reduce absorption. Once weekly therapy may enhance compliance.
6. If dietary intake is inadequate, take calcium with vitamin D supplements.
7. Do not drink alcoholic beverages or smoke while taking this drug.

# Rx: Uroxatral.

**CLASSIFICATION(S):** Treat benign prostatic hypertrophy (alpha-1 receptor antagonist)

**USES:** Signs and symptoms of benign prostatic hyperplasia (BPH).

**ACTION/KINETICS:** Selective antagonist of postsynaptic alpha-1 adrenergic receptors located in various areas of the prostate. Blockade of these receptors causes relaxation of smooth muscle in the bladder neck and prostate, resulting in an improvement in urine flow and a reduction in symptoms of BPH. **Maximum levels:** 8 hr after multiple dosing. Absorption is 50% lower under fasting conditions; thus, take immediately following a meal. Metabolites and unchanged drug are excreted in the feces (69%) and urine (24%). **t½, elimination:** 10 hr.

**SIDE EFFECTS:** Dizziness, headache, fatigue, URTI.

---

**DOSAGE: Tablets, Extended-Release**

*Benign prostatic hyperplasia.*

**Adults:** 10 mg daily immediately after the same meal each day.

---

**NEED TO KNOW**

1. Do not use with itraconazole, ketoconazole, ritonavir, other alpha-adrenergic blockers, or another potent inhibitor of CYP3A4.
2. Use with caution in clients with symptomatic hypotension or who have had a hypotensive response to other drugs. Use with caution in severe renal insufficiency.
3. Do not chew/crush tablets.
4. May experience drop in BP with sudden change in position; change positions slowly and use caution.
5. Report lack of response, chest pain, or adverse side effects. Keep all follow up visits to evaluate drug response.

## Allopurinol

(al-oh-**PYOUR**-ih-nohl)

**Rx:** Aloprim for Injection, Zyloprim.

**CLASSIFICATION(S):** Antigout drug

**USES: PO:** Primary or secondary gout (acute attacks, tophi, joint destruction, nephropathy, uric acid lithiasis). **PO and IV:** Clients with leukemia, lymphoma, or other malignancies in whom drug therapy causes elevations of serum and urinary uric acid. Recurrent calcium oxalate calculi where daily uric acid excretion exceeds 800 mg/day in males and 750 mg/day in females.

**ACTION/KINETICS:** Allopurinol and its major metabolite, oxipurinol, are potent inhibitors of xanthine oxidase, an enzyme involved in the synthesis of uric acid. Results in decreased uric acid levels. Also allopurinol increases reutilization of xanthine and hypoxanthine for synthesis of nucleotide and nucleic acid. The resultant increases in nucleotides cause a negative feedback to inhibit synthesis of purines and a decrease in uric acid levels.

**Peak plasma levels, after PO:** 1.5 hr for allopurinol and 4.5 hr for oxipurinol. **Onset, after PO:** 2–3 days. **t½, after PO** (allopurinol); 1–3 hr; **t½** (oxipurinol): 12–30 hr. **Peak serum levels after PO, allopurinol:** 2–3 mcg/mL; **oxipurinol:** 5–6.5 mcg/mL (up to 50 mcg/mL in clients with impaired renal function). Well absorbed from GI tract, metabolized in liver, excreted in urine and feces (20%).

**SIDE EFFECTS:** Rash, N&V, renal failure/insufficiency. STEVENS-JOHNSON SYNDROME, TOXIC EPIDERMAL NECROLYSIS, STATUS EPILEPTICUS, HEPATIC NECROSIS, LIVER FAILURE, CARDIORESPIRATORY ARREST, HEART FAILURE, HEMORRHAGE, STROKE, SEPTIC SHOCK, VENTRICULAR FIBRILLATION, ARDS, RESPIRATORY FAILURE, PULMONARY EMBOLUS.

## DOSAGE: IV Infusion

*Lower serum uric acid in leukemia, lymphoma, or solid malignancies.*

**Adults:** 200–400 mg/m$^2$/day, to a maximum of 600 mg/day.

**DOSAGE: Tablets**

*Gout/hyperuricemia.*
**Adults:** 200–300 mg/day for mild gout and 400–600 mg/day for moderately severe tophaceous gout, not to exceed 800 mg/day. Minimum effective dose: 100–200 mg/day.

*Prevention of uric acid nephropathy during vigorous treatment of neoplasms.*
**Adults:** 600–800 mg/day for 2–3 days (with high fluid intake).

*Prophylaxis of flare-up of acute gouty attacks.*
**Adults, initial:** 100 mg/day; increase by 100 mg at weekly intervals to achieve serum uric acid level of 6 mg/100 mL or less.

*Recurrent calcium oxalate calculi.*
**Adults:** 200–300 mg/day in one or more doses (dose may be adjusted according to urinary levels of uric acid).

---

**NEED TO KNOW**

1. Use with caution in clients with liver or renal disease.
2. Keep urine slightly alkaline to prevent uric acid stone formation.
3. Reduce PO dose as follows in impaired renal function: creatinine clearance ($C_{CR}$) less than 10 mL/min: 100 mg 3 times per week; $C_{CR}$ 10 mL/min: 100 mg every other day; $C_{CR}$ 20 mL/min: 100 mg/day; $C_{CR}$ 40 mL/min: 150 mg/day; $C_{CR}$ 60 mL/min: 200 mg/day.
4. Give daily IV dose as a single infusion or in equally divided infusions at 6-, 8-, or 12-hr intervals at concentration not to exceed 6 mg/mL.
5. Take with food or immediately after meals to lessen gastric irritation. Consume at least 10–12 8-oz glasses of fluid per day to prevent stone formation.
6. When using IV, ensure sufficient fluid intake to yield a daily urinary output of at least 2 L; maintain neutral, or preferably, a slightly alkaline urine (pH greater than 7).
7. Monitor weight with N&V or other signs of gastric irritation; report persistent weight loss.

8. Avoid caffeine and alcoholic beverages; decreases allopurinol effect.

---

## Alprazolam
(al-**PRAYZ**-oh-lam)

**D**

**Rx:** Alprazolam Extended-Release, Alprazolam Intensol, Niravam, Xanax, Xanax XR, **C-IV.**

---

**CLASSIFICATION(S):** Antianxiety drug, benzodiazepine
**USES: Immediate-Release Tablets, Orally Disintegrating Tablets and Intensol:** (1) Anxiety. (2) Anxiety associated with depression with or without agoraphobia. **Immediate- and Extended-Release Tablets, Orally Disintegrating Tablets:** Panic disorder with or without agoraphobia.
**ACTION/KINETICS:** Reduces anxiety by increasing or facilitating the inhibitory neurotransmitter activity of GABA. The skeletal muscle relaxant effect may be due to enhancement of GABA-mediated presynaptic inhibition at the spinal level as well as in the brain stem reticular formation. **Onset:** Intermediate. **Peak plasma levels:** PO, 8–37 ng/mL after 1–2 hr. $t^{1/2}$: 12–15 hr. Sublingual absorption is as rapid as PO use. Metabolized to alpha-hydroxyalprazolam, an active metabolite. $t^{1/2}$: 12–15 hr. Excreted in urine.
**SIDE EFFECTS:** Drowsiness, ataxia, confusion.

---

**DOSAGE: Oral Solution; Tablets, Immediate-Release; Tablets, Oral Disintegrating**

*Anxiety disorders.*

**Adults, initial:** 0.25–0.5 mg 3 times per day; **then,** titrate to needs of client at intervals of 3–4 days in increments of no more than 1 mg/day, with total daily dosage not to exceed 4 mg. **In elderly or debilitated, initial:** 0.25 mg 2–3 times per day; **then,** adjust dosage to needs of client.

lease; Tablets, Oral Disintegrating

*Panic disorders (use Niravam, Xanax, Xanax XR).*

**Adults, initial: Immediate-Release Tablets, Oral Disintegrating Tablets:** 0.5 mg 3 times per day; increase dose as needed, every 3–4 days in increments of no more than 1 mg/day up to a maximum of 10 mg/day (mean dose: 5–6 mg/day). **Extended-Release Tablets: Adults, initial:** 0.5–1 mg once daily. **Total daily dose:** 3–6 mg/day.

*Agoraphobia with social phobia.*

**Adults:** 2–8 mg/day.

## NEED TO KNOW

1. Do not use with itraconazole or ketoconazole.
2. Do not decrease daily dose more than 0.5 mg over 3 days if therapy terminated or dose decreased.
3. Reduce dosage in elderly and debilitated clients. Starting dose of immediate-release and intensol is 0.25 mg given 2 or 3 times per day. Increase dose gradually if needed. For extended-release tablets, begin with 0.5 mg once a day; gradually increase if needed and tolerated.
4. Avoid abrupt discontinuation due to the possibility of withdrawal. When discontinuing therapy or decreasing the daily dose, reduce dosage gradually.
5. Do not chew, crush, or break the extended-release tablet.
6. Mix Intensol oral solution with liquids or semi-solid foods such as water, juices, soda or soda-like beverages, applesauce, and puddings. Use the calibrated dropper provided.
7. May take tablets with milk or food to decrease GI upset.
8. Avoid activities that require mental alertness; may cause drowsiness.
9. Use support devices as needed, especially at night; elderly tend to become confused. Store drug away from bedside to prevent overdose.
10. Avoid smoking, alcohol consumption, or any other CNS depressants without provider approval.

# Amlodipine
(am-**LOH**-dih-peen)
**Rx:** Amvaz, Norvasc.

**C**

**CLASSIFICATION(S):** Calcium channel blocker
**USES:** (1) Hypertension alone or in combination with other antihypertensives. (2) Chronic stable angina alone or in combination with other antianginal drugs. (3) Vasospastic (Prinzmetal's variant) angina alone or in combination with other antianginal drugs.
**ACTION/KINETICS:** Inhibits influx of calcium through the cell membrane, resulting in a depression of automaticity and conduction velocity in cardiac muscle. Decreases SA and AV conduction and prolongs AV node effective and functional refractory periods.
**Peak plasma levels:** 6–12 hr. **t½, elimination:** 30–50 hr. 90% metabolized in the liver to inactive metabolites; 10% excreted unchanged in the urine.
**SIDE EFFECTS:** Edema, palpitations, dizziness/lightheadedness, headache, fatigue/lethargy, flushing. *CARDIAC FAILURE.*

## DOSAGE: Tablets

*Hypertension.*
  **Adults, usual, individualized:** 5 mg/day, up to a maximum of 10 mg/day. Titrate the dose over 7–14 days.

*Chronic stable or vasospastic angina.*
  **Adults:** 5–10 mg, using the lower dose for elderly clients and those with hepatic insufficiency. Most clients require 10 mg.

## NEED TO KNOW

1. Use with caution in clients with CHF and in those with impaired hepatic function or reduced hepatic blood flow.
2. Elderly clients, small/fragile clients, or those with hepatic insufficiency may be started on 2.5 mg/day.
3. Can be given safely with ACEI, beta-blockers, nitrates (long-acting), nitroglycerin (sublingual), or thiazides.

upset. Avoid grapefruit juice; increases drug concentrations.
5. Report S&S of chest pain, SOB, dizziness, swelling of extremities, irregular pulse, or altered vision immediately.
6. Use caution, may experience lightheadedness or dizziness.

---

## Anakinra
(**an**-ah-**KIN**-rah)

**B**

**Rx:** Kineret.

**CLASSIFICATION(S):** Antiarthritic

**USES:** Decrease signs and symptoms and slow the progression of structural damage in moderate-to-severe active rheumatoid arthritis in clients who have failed 1 or more disease modifying antirheumatic drugs (DMARD). Can be used alone or with DMARDs (except tissue necrosis factor blocking drugs).

**ACTION/KINETICS:** Interleukin-1 (IL-1) production is induced by inflammation. IL-1 degrades cartilage due to its induction of the rapid loss of proteoglycans, as well as stimulation of bone resorption. Anakinra blocks the biologic activity of IL-1 by competitively inhibiting IL-1 binding to the interleukin-1 type I receptor found in many tissues and organs. Thus, symptoms of rheumatoid arthritis improve. **Maximum plasma levels:** 3–7 hr. **t½, terminal:** 4–6 hr. Plasma clearance decreased 70–75% in those with severe or end-stage renal disease.

**SIDE EFFECTS:** Injection site reaction, worsening of RA, URTI, headache, nausea, diarrhea, sinusitis, arthralgia, flu-like symptoms, abdominal pain.

---

**DOSAGE: SC**

*Rheumatoid arthritis.*
**Adults:** 100 mg/day.

---

**NEED TO KNOW**
1. Associated with an increased incidence of serious infections

(especially when used with etanercept). Safety and efficacy have not been determined in immunosuppressed clients, in those with chronic infections, or when used with blocking agents.
2. Elderly clients may be more sensitive to the drug effects.
3. Give only one dose per day (i.e., entire contents of 1 prefilled glass syringe). Discard any unused portion; no preservative in product.
4. Inject anakinra daily, at same time each day, into the tissues as prescribed.
5. Injection site reactions may occur usually lasting 1–2 weeks. Rotate sites, report any pain, inflammation, bruising at sites.
6. Stop drug and report if any infection suspected.

---

## Anastrozole            D
(an-**AS**-troh-zohl)
**Rx:** Arimidex.

**CLASSIFICATION(S):** Antineoplastic, hormone
**USES:** (1) First-line treatment in postmenopausal women with advanced or locally advanced breast cancer whose disease is hormone receptor positive or hormone receptor unknown. (2) Advanced breast cancer in postmenopausal women with progression of the disease following tamoxifen therapy. (3) Adjuvant treatment of postmenopausal early breast cancer that is hormone receptor positive.
**ACTION/KINETICS:** Growth of many breast cancers is due to stimulation of estrogen receptors by estrogens. In postmenopausal women the main source of circulating estrogen is conversion of androstenedione to estrone by aromatase in peripheral tissues with further conversion to estradiol. Anastrozole is a nonsteroidal aromatase inhibitor that significantly decreases serum estradiol levels. Well absorbed from the GI tract; food does not affect the extent of absorption. **t½, terminal:** About 50 hr in postmenopaus-

al women. Metabolized by the liver and both unchanged drug (about 10%) and metabolites are excreted through the urine.

**SIDE EFFECTS:** GI disturbances, hot flashes, vasodilation, nausea, asthenia, back pain, pain, peripheral edema, bone pain, increased cough, dyspnea, headache. *VENOUS THROMBOEMBOLIC EVENTS, DVT EVENTS, ISCHEMIC CV EVENT, MI, STEVENS-JOHNSON SYNDROME (RARE).*

---

## DOSAGE: Tablets

*First-line treatment of advanced or locally advanced breast cancer. Advanced breast cancer following tamoxifen therapy. Adjuvant treatment of early breast cancer.*

**Adults:** 1 mg daily.

---

**NEED TO KNOW**

1. For first-line therapy, continue treatment until tumor regression evident.
2. For adjuvant treatment of early breast cancer, treatment is long-term (up to 5 years).
3. Take as directed at same time daily; usually on empty stomach 1 hr before or 3 hr after meals. Consume fluids; ensure adequate hydration.
4. Report unusual side effects, increased SOB/pain. May experience rash, hot flashes, itching, and skin lesions.

---

**Atenolol**
(ah-**TEN**-oh-lohl)                                     **C**
**Rx:** Tenormin.

**CLASSIFICATION(S):** Beta-adrenergic blocking agent
**USES:** (1) Hypertension (either alone or with other antihypertensives such as thiazide diuretics). (2) Long-term treatment of angina pectoris due to coronary atherosclerosis. (3) Acute MI.
**ACTION/KINETICS:** Combines reversibly with beta-adrenergic receptors to block the response to sympathetic nerve impulses, circulating catecholamines, or adrenergic drugs. Predominantly

beta-1 blocking activity. Has no membrane stabilizing activity or intrinsic sympathomimetic activity. **Peak blood levels:** 2–4 hr. t½: 6–9 hr. 50% eliminated unchanged in the feces. Geriatric clients have a higher plasma level than younger clients and a total clearance value of about 50% less.

**SIDE EFFECTS:** Dizziness, fatigue, nausea, bradycardia, hypotension, vertigo.

## DOSAGE: Tablets

*Hypertension.*
   **Adults, initial:** 50 mg/day, either alone or with diuretics; if response is inadequate, 100 mg/day. Doses higher than 100 mg/day will not produce further beneficial effects. Maximum effects usually seen within 1–2 weeks.

*Angina.*
   **Adults, initial:** 50 mg/day; if maximum response is not seen in 1 week, increase dose to 100 mg/day (some clients require 200 mg/day).

## DOSAGE: IV

*Acute myocardial infarction.*
   **Adults, initial:** 5 mg over 5 min followed by a second 5-mg dose 10 min later. Begin treatment as soon as possible after client arrives at the hospital. In clients who tolerate the full 10-mg dose, give a 50-mg tablet 10 min after the last IV dose followed by another 50-mg dose 12 hr later. **Then,** 100 mg/day or 50 mg twice a day for 6–9 days (or until discharge from the hospital).

## NEED TO KNOW

1. For IV use, may be diluted in NaCl injection, dextrose injection, or both.
2. If any question in using IV atenolol, eliminate IV administration and use tablets, 100 mg once daily or 50 mg twice a day for 7 or more days.

3. Take at same time each day. May take with food if GI upset occurs.
4. May mask symptoms of low blood sugar in those with diabetes.
5. With angina, do not stop abruptly; may cause anginal attack.
6. May enhance sensitivity to cold, dress accordingly.

## Atorvastatin calcium
(ah-**TORE**-vah-**stah**-tin)

**Rx:** Lipitor.

**CLASSIFICATION(S):** Antihyperlipidemic, HMG-CoA reductase inhibitor

**USES:** (1) Adjunct to diet to decrease elevated total and LDL cholesterol, Apo-B, and triglyceride levels and to increase HDL cholesterol in primary hypercholesterolemia (including heterozygous familial and nonfamilial) and mixed dyslipidemia (including Fredrickson type IIa and IIb). (2) Adjunct to other lipid-lowering treatments to reduce total and LDL cholesterol in homozygous familial hypercholesterolemia. (3) Primary dysbetalipoproteinemia (Fredrickson type III) in those who do not respond adequately to diet. (4) Adjunct to diet to treat elevated serum triglyceride levels (Fredrickson type IV). (5) Reduce the risk of nonfatal MI, fatal and nonfatal stroke, revascularization procedures, hospitalization for CHF, and angina in clients with clinically evident coronary heart disease. (6) Reduce the risk of MI and stroke and the risk for revascularization procedures and angina in adults without clinically evident coronary heart disease but with multiple risk factors for coronary heart disease, including age, smoking, hypertension, low HDL-C, or a family history of early coronary heart disease. (7) Reduce the risk of stroke and MI in type 2 diabetics who show no evidence of coronary heart disease but with other risk factors, including retinopathy, albuminuria, smoking, or hypertension.

**ACTION/KINETICS:** Competitively inhibits HMG-CoA reductase; this enzyme catalyzes the early rate-limiting step in the synthesis

13

of cholesterol. Decreases cholesterol, triglycerides, VLDL, and LDL and increases HDL. Undergoes first-pass metabolism by CYP3A4 enzymes to active metabolites. $t\frac{1}{2}$: 14 hr. Metabolized in the liver to active metabolites. Decreases in LDL cholesterol range from 35–40% (10 mg/day) to 50–60% (80 mg/day). Less than 2% excreted in the urine.

**SIDE EFFECTS:** Headache, asthenia, abdominal pain/cramps, infection, diarrhea, sinusitis, pharyngitis, myalgia, arthralgia, back pain, rash/pruritus, flu syndrome.

## DOSAGE: Tablets

*Hypercholesterolemia (heterozygous familial and non-familial) and mixed dyslipidemia (Fredrickson types IIa and IIb).*

**Adults, initial:** 10–20 mg once daily (40 mg/day for those who require more than a 45% reduction in LDL cholesterol); **then,** a dose range of 10–80 mg once daily may be used. Individualize therapy according to goal of therapy and response.

*Homozygous familial hypercholesterolemia.*

**Adults, initial:** 10–80 mg/day. Used as an adjunct to other lipid-lowering treatments, such as LDL apheresis.

*Prophylaxis of CV disease.*

**Adults:** 10 mg/day.

## NEED TO KNOW

1. Give as single dose at any time of the day, with or without food.
2. For additive effect, may be used in combination with a bile acid binding resin. Do not use atorvastatin with fibrates.
3. Continue dietary restrictions of saturated fat and cholesterol, regular exercise and weight loss in the overall goal of lowering cholesterol levels. See dietician for additional dietary recommendations.
4. Report any unexplained muscle pain, weakness, or tenderness, especially if accompanied by fever or malaise.
5. Use UV protection (i.e., sunglasses, sunscreens, clothing/hat)

to prevent photosensitivity. Avoid prolonged exposure to direct or artificial sunlight.

# Budesonide   **B**
(byou-DES-oh-nyd)
**Rx: Capsules**: Entocort EC. **Inhalation**: Pulmicort Flexhaler, Pulmicort Respules, Pulmicort Turbuhaler. **Intranasal**: Rhinocort Aqua.

**CLASSIFICATION(S):** Glucocorticoid

**USES:** (1) **Entocort EC:** Treatment and maintenance (up to 3 months) of clinical remission of mild-to-moderate active Crohn's disease involving the ileum and/or ascending colon. (2) **Pulmicort Flexhaler:** Prophylaxis and maintenance treatment of asthma, including those requiring PO corticosteroid therapy for asthma. (3) **Pulmicort Turbuhaler:** Maintenance treatment of asthma as prophylaxis in adults; also for those requiring oral corticosteroid therapy for asthma. (4) **Rhinocort Aqua:** Treat symptoms of seasonal or perennial allergic rhinitis in adults.

**ACTION/KINETICS:** Exerts a direct local anti-inflammatory effect with minimal systemic effects when used intranasally. Exceeding the recommended dose may result in suppression of hypothalamic-pituitary-adrenal function. **Onset, nasal spray:** 10 hr. **t½:** 2–3 hr. Rapidly metabolized by CYP3A liver enzymes. Excreted through both urine and feces.

**SIDE EFFECTS: Inhalation Powder:** Headache, URTI, flu-like symptoms, sinusitis, pharyngitis, back pain/pain, bronchospasm, cough, epistaxis. **Inhalation Suspension:** URTI, rhinitis, nasal congestion, otitis media/ear infection, epistaxis. **Oral:** Headache, tremor, rash, acne, fainting. **For all routes:** BRONCHIAL ASTHMA, IMMEDIATE AND DELAYED HYPERSENSITIVITY REACTIONS.

## DOSAGE: Capsules
*Crohn's disease.*

**Adults:** 9 mg once daily in the a.m. for up to 8 weeks. If the disease recurs, another 8-week course may be given. Once symptoms are controlled, give 6 mg once daily for maintenance of clinical remission for up to 3 months. If symptom control is still maintained at 3 months, attempt to taper to complete cessation.

## DOSAGE: Pulmicort Turbuhaler

*Prevention or treatment of asthma.*

**Adults, initial, if previous therapy was bronchodilators alone: 200–400 mcg twice a day, not to exceed 400 mcg twice a day. Initial, if previous therapy was inhaled corticosteroids for well controlled mild to moderate asthma: 200–400 mcg (1–2 inhalations) once daily either in the morning or evening. Do not exceed 800 mcg twice a day. Initial, if previous therapy was oral corticosteroids: 400–800 mcg twice a day, not to exceed 800 mcg twice a day.**

## DOSAGE: Aqua Nasal Spray (Rhinocort Aqua)

*Seasonal and perennial allergic rhinitis.*

**Adults, initial:** 1 spray/nostril (64 mcg/day) once daily. **Maximum:** 4 sprays/nostril (256 mcg) once daily. After the maximum effect is obtained, reduce the maintenance dose to the smallest amount required to control symptoms.

## NEED TO KNOW

1. Do not use for acute or life-threatening asthma attacks, including status asthmaticus.
2. Use with caution in clients already on alternate-day corticosteroids (e.g., prednisone); in clients with active or quiescent tuberculosis infections of the respiratory tract, or in untreated fungal, bacterial infections or systemic viral infections; or ocular herpes simplex.
3. Turbuhaler does not require spacer; delivers about twice the amount of drug per inhalation to the airway as metered dose inhalers.

4. Rinse mouth and equipment thoroughly after each use to prevent oral fungal infections.
5. Maximum benefit usually not seen for 3–7 days, although a decrease in symptoms can be seen within 24 hr. Report if no improvement within 3 weeks.
6. Shake canister well before administering. Store valve down and away from areas of high humidity. Once Al pouch opened, use/discard within 6 months. Prime unit before use with Pulmicort Turbuhaler.
7. Prior to using nasal spray gently shake container and prime the pump by actuating 8 times. If not used for 2 consecutive days, reprime with 1 spray or until a fine mist appears. If not used for more than 14 days, rinse the applicator and reprime with 2 sprays or until a fine mist appears.
8. Report chest pain, lower extremity swelling, severe headaches, respiratory infections, or increased bruising/bleeding.

---

## Bupropion hydrochloride    **B**
(byou-**PROH**-pee-on)

**Rx:** Budeprion SR, Budeprion XL, Wellbutrin, Wellbutrin SR, Wellbutrin XL, Zyban.

**CLASSIFICATION(S):** Antidepressant, miscellaneous; smoking deterrent (Zyban)

**USES:** (1) Treatment of major depressive episodes (immediate-release, extended-release, and sustained-release). (2) Major depressive episodes in those with a history of seasonal affective disorder (Budeprion XL). (3) Aid to stop smoking (Zyban only); may be combined with a nicotine transdermal system.

**ACTION/KINETICS:** Its action is believed to be mediated by noradrenergic and/or dopaminergic mechanisms. Exerts moderate anticholinergic and sedative effects, but only slight orthostatic hypotension. **Peak plasma levels, Wellbutrin SR and Zyban:** 3 hr; **peak plasma levels, Wellbutrin XL:** 5 hr. **t½, terminal, immediate-release:** 8–24 hr. **Time to steady state:** Within 8 days. Significantly metabolized by a first-pass effect through the liver to both active and inactive metabolites. Can induce drug-metabolizing enzymes. Excreted through both the urine (87%) and the feces (10%).

**SIDE EFFECTS:** Agitation, anxiety, constipation, dizziness, headache/migraine, insomnia, tremor, sedation, excessive sweating, anorexia, dry mouth, N&V. *SEIZURES, SUICIDAL IDEATION, STROKE.*

## DOSAGE: Tablets, Immediate-Release

*Antidepressant.*

**Adults, initial:** 100 mg in the a.m. and p.m. for the first 3 days; **then,** 100 mg 3 times per day, given in the morning, midday, and in the evening (6 hr should elapse between doses). If no response is observed after 4 weeks or more, the dose may be increased to a maximum of 450 mg/day with individual doses not to exceed 150 mg. **Maintenance:** Lowest dose to control depression.

## DOSAGE: Tablets, Extended-Release (XL)

*Antidepressant, seasonal affective disorder.*

**Adults, initial:** 150 mg/day in the morning; **maintenance:** 300 mg/day in the morning. Maintenance dose may be increased to 450 mg/day in the morning if no improvement seen after several weeks of 300 mg/day. There should be an interval of at least 24 hr between successive doses. Periodically assess to determine the need for maintenance treatment and the appropriate dose for such treatment.

## DOSAGE: Tablets, Sustained-Release (SR)

*Antidepressant.*

**Adults, initial:** 150 mg once daily in the a.m. If 150 mg is tolerated, increase to 300 mg/day given as 150 mg twice a day as early as day 4 of dosing. Allow 8 or more hr between successive doses. Do not exceed a daily dose of 400 mg given as 200 mg twice a day in clients where no clinical improvement was noted after several weeks of 300 mg/day. **Maintenance:**

Periodically assess to determine the need for maintenance treatment and the appropriate dose for such treatment.

---

## DOSAGE: Zyban

*Smoking deterrent.*

**Adults, initial:** 150 mg/day for the first 3 days; **then,** 150 mg twice a day for 7–12 weeks (up to 6 months). Do not exceed doses of 300 mg/day. Eight hours or more should elapse between successive doses.

---

### NEED TO KNOW

1. Do not use with a MAOI.
2. Do not use in clients undergoing abrupt discontinuation of alcohol and sedatives, including benzodiazepines.
3. Use with extreme caution in clients with cranial trauma, with drugs that lower the seizure threshold, and situations that might cause seizures.
4. Adults with major depressive disease may show worsening of their depression and/or the emergence of suicidal ideation and behavior or unusual changes in behavior, whether or not they are taking antidepressants.
5. Use with caution and in lower doses in clients with liver or kidney disease and in those with a recent history of MI or unstable heart disease.
6. The risk of seizures may be minimized by using the following guidelines: **For Bupropion IR:** Do not exceed a total daily dose of 450 mg. The daily dose is given 3 times per day with at least 6 hr between successive doses, with each single dose not to exceed 150 mg. The rate of dose increase is very gradual. **For Wellbutrin SR:** Do not exceed a total daily dose of 400 mg. The daily dose is given twice daily. The rate of dose increase is gradual. No single dose should exceed 200 mg. **For Bupropion XL:** Do not exceed a total daily dose of 450 mg. The rate of dose increase is gradual. **For Zyban:** Do not exceed a total daily dose of 300 mg. The recommended daily

dose for most clients is 300 mg/day given as 150 mg twice a day. No single dose should exceed 150 mg.

7. May experience changes in taste perception; may result in appetite/weight loss.

8. Dizziness may occur. Do not arise from lying position suddenly. If dizziness occurs during the day, sit until it subsides. May cause drowsiness, hyperactivity, GI upset, diarrhea, constipation, dry mouth. Avoid activities that require mental alertness until effects realized.

---

## Celecoxib C
(**sell**-ah-**KOX**-ihb)
**Rx:** Celebrex.

**CLASSIFICATION(S):** Nonsteroidal anti-inflammatory, COX-2 inhibitor

**USES:** (1) Relief of signs and symptoms of rheumatoid arthritis and osteoarthritis in adults. (2) Acute pain in adults. (3) Relief of signs and symptoms of ankylosing spondylitis. (4) Reduce the number of adenomatous colorectal polyps in familial adenomatous polyposis, as an adjunct to usual care.

**ACTION/KINETICS:** Inhibits prostaglandin synthesis, primarily by inhibiting cyclo-oxygenase-2 (COX-2), thus decreasing inflammation. Causes fewer GI complications, such as bleeding and perforation, compared with other NSAIDs. **Peak plasma levels:** 3 hr. **t½, terminal:** 11 hr when fasting; low solubility prolongs absorption. Metabolized in the liver to inactive compounds; excreted in the urine (27%) and feces (57%).

**SIDE EFFECTS:** Abdominal pain/cramps, diarrhea, nausea, dyspepsia/indigestion, URTI. *GI HEMORRHAGE.*

---

**DOSAGE: Capsules**

*Osteoarthritis.*

    **Adults:** 100 mg twice a day or 200 mg as a single dose.

*Rheumatoid arthritis.*

**Adults:** 100–200 mg twice a day.

*Anklyosing spondylitis.*

**Adults:** 200 mg daily either as a single dose or divided into 2 doses. If no effect is seen after 6 weeks, a trial of 400 mg/day may be beneficial.

*Acute pain.*

**Adults, day 1, Initial:** 400 mg; **then,** an additional 200 mg, if needed on day 1. On subsequent days, 200 mg 2 times per day, as needed.

*Familial adenomatous polyposis.*

**Adults:** 400 mg twice a day with food. Continue usual medical care (e.g., endoscopic surveillance, surgery).

---

**NEED TO KNOW**

1. Celecoxib may cause an increased risk of serious CV thrombotic events, MI, and stroke, which can be fatal. All NSAIDs may have a similar risk.
2. Celecoxib is contraindicated for the treatment of perioperative pain in the setting of coronary artery bypass graft.
3. NSAIDs, including celecoxib, cause an increased risk of serious GI adverse effects, including bleeding, ulceration, and perforation of the stomach or intestines, which can be fatal.
4. Reduce daily dose by about 50% in clients with moderate impaired hepatic function (Child-Pugh class B).
5. For those unable to swallow capsules, the contents of a celecoxib capsule can be added to a level teaspoon of applesauce; ingest immediately with water.
6. Take with food; decreases stomach upset.
7. Avoid prolonged exposure to direct or artificial sunlight.
8. Report unusual/persistent side effects, including dyspepsia, abdominal pain, dizziness, changes in stool/skin color.

## Ciprofloxacin hydrochloride

C

(sip-row-**FLOX**-ah-sin)

**Rx:** Ciloxan Ophthalmic, Cipro, Cipro I.V., Cipro XR, Proquin XR.

**CLASSIFICATION(S):** Antibiotic, fluoroquinolone

**USES: Immediate Release (IR) Tablets and Oral Suspension.** (1) Acute sinusitis. (2) Acute uncomplicated cystitis in women. (3) Chronic bacterial prostatitis. (4) UTIs. (5) Bone and joint infections. (6) With metronidazole for complicated intra-abdominal infections. (7) Infectious diarrhea. (8) Lower respiratory tract infections. (9) Acute exacerbations of chronic bronchitis. (10) Skin and skin structure infections. (11) Typhoid fever (enteric fever). (12) Uncomplicated cervical and urethral gonorrhea. **Immediate-Release (IR) Tablets, IV, and Oral Suspension.** Reduce the incidence or progression of disease following exposure to aerosolized *Bacillus anthracis.* **Extended-Release (ER) Tablets Only.** (1) Uncomplicated UTIs. (2) Complicated UTIs (except Proquin XR). **IV.** (1) Acute sinusitis. (2) Chronic bacterial prostatitis. (3) UTIs. (4) Bone and joint infections. (5) With metronidazole for complicated intra-abdominal infections. (6) Acute exacerbations of chronic bronchitis. (7) Nosocomial pneumonia. (8) With piperacillin sodium as empirical therapy for febrile neutopenic clients. (9) Skin and skin structure infections. **Ocular Infections.** Superficial ocular infections involving the conjunctiva or cornea. **Ophthalmic Ointment.** Bacterial conjunctivitis. **Ophthalmic Solution.** (1) Corneal ulcers. (2) Conjunctivitis.

**ACTION/KINETICS:** Interferes with DNA gyrase and topoisomerase IV. DNA gyrase is an enzyme needed for replication, transcription, and repair of bacterial DNA. Topoisomerase IV plays a key role in the partitioning of chromosomal DNA during bacterial cell division. Effective against both gram-positive and gram-negative organisms. Rapidly and well absorbed following PO administration. Food delays absorption of the drug. **Maximum serum lev-**

els: 2–4 mcg/mL 1–2 hr after dosing. **t½:** 4 hr for PO use and 5–6 hr for IV use. Avoid peak serum levels above 5 mcg/mL. About 40–50% of a PO dose and 50–70% of an IV dose is excreted unchanged in the urine.

**SIDE EFFECTS: After systemic use:** Headache, N&V, diarrhea, restlessness, rash. *INTESTINAL PERFORATION, ANGIOEDEMA, TOXIC EPIDERMAL NECROLYSIS, STEVENS-JOHNSON SYNDROME, MI, CEREBRAL THROMBOSIS, BRONCHOSPASM, PULMONARY EMBOLISM, EDEMA OF LARYNX OR LUNGS, AGRANULOCYTOSIS, HEPATIC NECROSIS.* **After ophthalmic use:** Irritation, burning, stinging, itching, inflammation.

---

**DOSAGE: Oral Suspension; Tablets, Extended-Release; Tablets, Immediate-Release**

*UTIs.*
> **Adults: Acute, uncomplicated infections:** 250 mg q 12 hr for 3 days or 500 mg once daily of extended-release tablets for 3 days. **Mild to moderate infections:** 250 mg q 12 hr for 7–14 days. **Severe/complicated infections:** 500 mg q 12 hr for 7–14 days or 1,000 mg once daily of extended-release tablets for 7–14 days.

*Pyelonephritis, acute uncomplicated.*
> **Adults:** 1,000 mg once daily of extended-release tablets for 7–14 days.

*Mild to moderate chronic bacterial prostatitis.*
> **Adults:** 500 mg q 12 hr for 28 days.

*Mild to moderate acute sinusitis.*
> **Adults:** 500 mg q 12 hr for 10 days.

*Urethral or cervical gonococcal infections, uncomplicated.*
> **Adults:** 250 mg in a single dose.

*Infectious diarrhea, mild to severe.*
> **Adults:** 500 mg q 12 hr for 5–7 days.

*Skin and skin structures, lower respiratory tract, bone and joint infections.*
> **Adults:** 500 mg (mild to moderate) to 750 mg (severe or com-

plicated) q 12 hr for 7–14 days (4–6 weeks for bone and joint infections).

*Intra-abdominal infections, complicated.*
   **Adults:** 500 mg q 12 hr for 7–14 days with metronidazole.

*Typhoid fever, mild to moderate.*
   **Adults:** 500 mg q 12 hr for 10 days.

*Inhalational anthrax (postexposure).*
   **Adults:** 500 mg q 12 hr for 60 days.

**DOSAGE: IV Infusion**

*UTIs.*
   **Adults:** 200 mg (mild to moderate) to 400 mg (severe or complicated) q 12 hr for 7–14 days.

*Skin and skin structures, lower respiratory tract, bone and joint infections.*
   **Adults: Mild to moderate infections:** 400 mg q 12 hr for 7–14 days. **Severe/complicated infections:** 400 mg q 8 hr for 7–14 days. Up to 4–6 weeks may be needed for bone and joint infections.

*Nosocomial pneumonia, mild to severe.*
   **Adults:** 400 mg q 8 hr for 10–14 days.

*Febrile neutropenic clients, empirical therapy, severe.*
   **Adults:** 400 mg q 8 hr with piperacillin, 50 mg/kg q 4 hr, not to exceed 24 grams/day, each for 7–14 days.

*Acute sinusitis, mild to moderate.*
   **Adults:** 400 mg q 12 hr for 10 days.

*Chronic bacterial prostatitis, mild to moderate.*
   **Adults:** 400 mg q 12 hr for 28 days.

*Intra-abdominal infections, complicated.*
   **Adults:** 400 mg q 12 hr for 7–14 days.

*Inhalational anthrax, postexposure.*
   **Adults:** 400 mg q 12 hr for 60 days.

*Disseminated gonococcal infections.*

**Adults:** 500 mg for 24–48 hr; after improvement begins, 500 mg PO 2 times per day for 7 days.

## DOSAGE: Ophthalmic Ointment

*Ocular infections.*

**Adults, initial:** Apply ½ in. ribbon to conjunctival sac 3 times per day for the first 2 days; **then,** ½ in. ribbon twice a day for the next 5 days.

## DOSAGE: Ophthalmic Solution

*Corneal ulcers.*

**Adults, first day, initial:** 2 gtt into the affected eye q 15 min for the first 6 hr; **then,** 2 gtt into the affected eye q 30 min for the remainder of the first day. **Second day:** 2 gtt into the affected eye hourly. **Third–Fourteenth day:** 2 gtt into the affected eye q 4 hr. If corneal re-epitheliazation has not occurred after 14 days, treatment may be continued.

*Conjunctivitis.*

**Adults, initial:** 1–2 gtt into the conjunctival sac q 2 hr while awake for 2 days; **then,** 1 or 2 gtt q 4 hr while awake for the next 5 days.

## NEED TO KNOW

1. Do not use ophthalmically in the presence of dendritic keratitis, varicella, vaccinia, and mycobacterial and fungal eye infections and after removal of foreign bodies from the cornea.
2. Dose must be reduced in those with a $C_{CR}$ less than 50 mL/min. The dose of immediate release tablets and suspension should be 250–500 mg q 12 hr if the $C_{CR}$ is 30–50 mL/min or 250–500 mg q 18 hr. For IV use, give 200–400 mg q 18–24 hr if the $C_{CR}$ is 5–29 mL/min. If the client is on hemodialysis or peritoneal dialysis, the dose of immediate-release and suspension should be 250–500 mg q 24 hr after dialysis.
3. Reconstitute IV solution dose to final concentration of 1–2 mg/mL and give over 60 min. To minimize discomfort/irritation, slowly infuse dilute solution into a large vein.
4. If started on IV ciprofloxacin, may be switched to tablets or

suspension when clinically indicated. Equivalent dosing regimens are as follows:
- 250 mg tablet q 12 hr = 200 mg IV q 12 hr.
- 500 mg tablet q 12 hr = 400 mg IV q 12 hr.
- 750 mg tablet q 12 hr = 400 mg IV q 8 hr.

5. XR tablets may be taken with meals that include milk; however, avoid with dairy products alone or with calcium-fortified products because of decreased absorption. A 2-hr window between substantial calcium intake (more than 800 mg) and dosing with XR tablets is recommended.
6. XR and IR tablets are not interchangeable.
7. Use caution; avoid sun exposure, direct or artificial sunlight may cause photosensitivity reaction.
8. Drink 2–3 L per day of fluids to keep the urine acidic and minimize risk of crystalluria.
9. Report any persistent joint/tendon pain (especially knee) or GI symptoms such as diarrhea, vomiting, or abdominal pain.

## Citalopram hydrobromide
(sigh-**TAL**-oh-pram)
**Rx:** Celexa.

**CLASSIFICATION(S):** Antidepressant, selective serotonin reuptake inhibitor
**USES:** Treatment of depression in those with DSM-IV category of major depressive disorder.
**ACTION/KINETICS:** Inhibits reuptake of serotonin into CNS neurons resulting in increased levels of serotonin in synapses. **Peak plasma levels:** 120–150 nmol/L after about 4 hr. **t½, terminal:** 35 hr. Half-life and AUC are increased in geriatric clients. **Steady state plasma levels:** About 1 week. Metabolized in the liver and excreted in the urine (20%) and feces (65%).
**SIDE EFFECTS:** Somnolence, insomnia, nausea, excessive sweat-

ing, dry mouth, tremor, loose stools/diarrhea. *SUICIDE IDEATION/AT-TEMPT, CARDIAC FAILURE, MI, CVA.*

**DOSAGE:** Oral Solution; Tablets; Tablets, Orally-Disintegrating
*Depression.*
    **Adults, initial:** 20 mg once daily in a.m. or p.m. with or without food. Increase dose in increments of 20 mg at intervals of no less than 1 week. Doses greater than 40 mg/day are not recommended. For the elderly or those with hepatic impairment, 20 mg/day is recommended; titrate to 40 mg/day only for nonresponders. Initial treatment is continued for 6 or 8 weeks. **Maintenance:** Up to 24 weeks following 6 or 8 weeks of initial treatment. Periodically re-evaluate the long-term usefulness of the drug if used for extended periods.

**NEED TO KNOW**
1. Use with caution in severe renal impairment (dosage adjustment not necessary), a history of seizure disorders, or in diseases or conditions that produce altered metabolism or hemodynamic responses.
2. Allow at least 14 days to elapse between discontinuation of a MAOI and initiation of citalopram or vice versa.
3. Take as directed, once daily, with or without food.
4. Avoid alcohol or other CNS depressants.

---

**Clopidogrel bisulfate**
(kloh-**PID**-oh-grel)
**Rx:** Plavix.

**B**

**CLASSIFICATION(S):** Antiplatelet drug
**USES:** (1) Non–ST-segment elevation acute coronary syndrome (unstable angina/non–Q-wave MI), including those who are to be managed medically and those who are to be managed with percutaneous coronary intervention (with or without stent) or coronary artery bypass graft. (2) To reduce the rate of death from any

cause and the rate of a combined end point of death, reinfarction, or stroke in those with ST-segment elevation acute MI. (3) To reduce the rate of a combined end point of new ischemic stroke (fatal or not), new MI (fatal or not), and other vascular death in those with a history of recent MI, recent stroke, or established peripheral arterial disease.

**ACTION/KINETICS:** Inhibits platelet aggregation by inhibiting binding of adenosine diphosphate (ADP) to its platelet receptor and subsequent ADP-mediative activation of glycoprotein GPIIb/IIIa complex. Also inhibits platelet aggregation caused by agonists other than ADP by blocking amplification of platelet activation by released ADP. Rapidly absorbed from GI tract; food does not affect bioavailability. **Peak plasma levels:** About 1 hr. Extensively metabolized in liver; about 50% excreted in urine and 46% in feces. **t½, elimination:** 8 hr.

**SIDE EFFECTS:** Skin/appendage disorders, headache, URTI, chest pain, flu-like symptoms. *INTRACRANIAL HEMORRHAGE, MAJOR/LIFE-THREATENING BLEEDING, RETROPERITONEAL HEMORRHAGE, HEMORRHAGE OF OPERATIVE WOUND, CARDIAC FAILURE, PULMONARY HEMORRHAGE, PERFORATED HEMORRHAGIC GASTRITIS, HEMORRHAGIC UPPER GI ULCER, PERFORATED GASTRIC ULCER, APLASTIC ANEMIA, PANCYTOPENIA, AGRANULOCYTOSIS, ANGIOEDEMA, STEVENS-JOHNSON SYNDROME, TOXIC EPIDERMAL NECROLYSIS, ACUTE RENAL FAILURE, ANAPHYLAXIS.*

**DOSAGE: Tablets**

*Acute coronary syndrome, non–ST-segment elevation.*

**Adults, initial:** Single 300 mg loading dose; **then,** 75 mg once daily. Initiate and continue aspirin (75–325 mg once daily). Many clients also receive heparin acutely.

*Acute coronary syndrome, ST-segment elevation.*

**Adults:** 75 mg once daily, given with aspirin, with or without thrombolytics. Clopidogrel may be initiated with or without a loading dose of 300 mg.

*Recent MI, stroke, or established peripheral arterial disease.*

**Adults:** 75 mg once daily.

## NEED TO KNOW

1. Use with caution in those at risk of increased bleeding from trauma, surgery, or other pathological conditions. Use with caution in severe impaired renal or hepatic function.
2. Drug interaction: Aspirin increases the risk of life-threatening or major bleeding events (e.g., intracranial and GI hemorrhage) in high-risk clients with recent ischemic stroke or TIAs.
3. Dosage adjustment not necessary for geriatric clients or with renal disease.
4. Take exactly as directed; may take without regard to food. Food will lessen chance of stomach upset.
5. May cause dizziness or drowsiness.
6. Avoid OTC agents especially aspirin, aspirin-containing products, or NSAIDs, unless prescribed.
7. Report any unusual bruising or bleeding; advise all providers of prescribed therapy.
8. Drug should be discontinued 7 days prior to elective surgery.

---

## Colchicine
### (KOHL-chih-seen)
**Rx:** Colchicine Tablets.

(oral use) **C**
(parenteral use) **D**

**CLASSIFICATION(S):** Antigout drug

**USES:** Prophylaxis and treatment of acute attacks of gout.

**ACTION/KINETICS:** May reduce the crystal-induced inflammation by reducing lactic acid production by leukocytes (resulting in a decreased deposition of sodium urate), by inhibiting leukocyte migration, and by reducing phagocytosis. May also inhibit the synthesis of kinins and leukotrienes. **t½, plasma:** 10–60 min. **Onset, IV:** 6–12 hr; **PO:** 12 hr. **Time to peak levels, PO:** 0.5–2 hr. It concentrates in leukocytes (t½, about 46 hr). Metabolized in the liver and mainly excreted in the feces with 10–20% excreted unchanged through the urine.

**SIDE EFFECTS:** N&V, diarrhea (may be severe), abdominal pain/cramps, dermatoses. *APLASTIC ANEMIA, AGRANULOCYTOSIS.*

## DOSAGE: Tablets

*Acute gouty arthritis.*

**Adults, usual:** 1.2 mg followed by 0.6 mg q 1–2 hr until pain is relieved or nausea, vomiting, or diarrhea occurs. **Total amount required:** 4–8 mg.

*Prophylaxis during intercritical periods.*

**Adults:** 0.6 mg/day for 3–4 days a week if the client has less than one attack per year or 0.6 mg/day if the client has more than one attack per year.

*Prophylaxis for surgical clients.*

**Adults:** 0.6 mg 3 times per day for 3 days before and 3 days after surgery.

## DOSAGE: IV only

*Acute attack of gout.*

**Adults, initial:** 2 mg; **then,** 0.5 mg q 6 hr until pain is relieved; give no more than 4 mg in a 24-hr period. If pain recurs, 1–2 mg/day may be given for several days; however, colchicine should not be given by any route for at least 7 days after a full course of IV therapy (i.e., 4 mg).

*Prophylaxis or maintenance of recurrent or chronic gouty arthritis.*

**Adults:** 0.5–1 mg 1–2 times per day. However, PO colchicine is preferred (usually with a uricosuric drug).

---

**NEED TO KNOW**

1. Do not use in presence of combined renal and hepatic disease.
2. Geriatric clients may be at greater risk of developing cumulative toxicity. Use with extreme caution for elderly, debilitated clients, especially in the presence of chronic renal, hepatic, GI, or CV disease.
3. Avoid extravasation; may cause tissue damage with resultant nerve damage.

4. Stop drug and report if N&V, or diarrhea develops; these are signs of toxicity.
5. Drug will not prevent the progression of this disease, only controls symptoms.
6. Consume 3–3.5 L/day of fluids to enhance crystal excretion.
7. NSAIDs may help with pain and inflammation; use as prescribed. Report any unusual bruising/bleeding, weakness, numbness or tingling, fatigue, rash, sore throat or fever.

## Conjugated estrogens and Medroxyprogesterone acetate  X
(**KON**-jyou-**gay**-ted **ES**- troh-jens, meh-**drox**-see-proh-**JESS**-ter-ohn)
**Rx:** PremPro, Premphase.

**CLASSIFICATION(S):** Sex hormones
**USES:** (1) Moderate to severe vasomotor symptoms associated with menopause in women with an intact uterus. (2) Vulvar and vaginal atrophy.
**ACTION/KINETICS:** Estrogens combine with receptors in the cytoplasm of cells, resulting in an increase in protein synthesis. During menopause, estrogens are used as replacement therapy. Medroxyprogesterone acetate reduces endometrial hyperplasia and may decrease the number of estrogen receptors. Estrogens are metabolized in the liver and excreted mainly in the urine. **Medroxyprogesterone acetate, maximum levels:** 1–2 hr. t$^{1}\!/_{2}$, **after PO:** 2–3 hr for first 6 hr; then, 8–9 hr.
**SIDE EFFECTS:** Abdominal/back pain, headache, nausea, infection, depression, breast pain.

---

**DOSAGE: Tablets**
*Vasomotor symptoms due to menopause, vulvar and vaginal atrophy, prevention of osteoporosis.*
   **Adults:** *PremPro:* One 0.625/2.5 mg tablet once daily. *Premphase:* One 0.625 mg conjugated estrogen tablet once daily

on days 1 to 14 and one 0.625/5 mg tablet once daily on days 15 to 28.

## NEED TO KNOW

1. Do not use in known or suspected cancer of the breast or estrogen-dependent neoplasia, undiagnosed abnormal genital bleeding, or active or past history of thrombophlebitis, thromboembolic disease, or stroke.
2. Use with caution in conditions aggravated by fluid retention, including asthma, epilepsy, migraine, and cardiac or renal dysfunction.
3. Estrogens may cause significant increases in plasma triglycerides that may cause pancreatitis and other complications in clients with familial defects of lipoprotein metabolism.
4. When used for treating vasomotor symptoms or vulvar and vaginal atrophy, re-evaluate every 3–6 months to assess treatment results.
5. Should not be used to prevent osteoporosis.

---

## Dalteparin sodium  B
(**DAL**-tih-**pair**-in)
**Rx:** Fragmin.

**CLASSIFICATION(S):** Anticoagulant, low molecular weight heparin
**USES:** (1) Prevent deep vein thrombosis (DVT) in clients undergoing hip replacement or abdominal surgery who are at risk for thromboembolic complications. (2) Prevent DVT in those who are at risk for thromboembolic complications (which may lead to pulmonary embolism) due to severely restricted mobility during acute illness. (3) Prevent ischemic complications due to blood clot formation in life-threatening unstable angina and non-Q-wave MI in clients coadministered aspirin. (4) Extended treatment of symptomatic venous thromboembolism (proximal deep vein thrombo-

sis and/or pulmonary embolism) to reduce the occurrence of venous thromboembolism in clients with cancer.

**ACTION/KINETICS: Peak plasma levels:** 4 hr. t½, **SC:** 3–5 hr. t½ increased in those with chronic renal insufficiency requiring hemodialysis.

**SIDE EFFECTS:** Hematomas (injection site, wound), significant bleeding, pruritus/rash, hematuria, allergic reaction, fever, injection site reactions. *ANAPHYLAXIS.*

---

## DOSAGE: SC Only

*Prevention of DVT in abdominal surgery.*

**Adults:** 2,500 international units each day starting 1–2 hr prior to surgery and repeated once daily for 5–10 days postoperatively. **High-risk clients:** 5,000 international units the night before surgery and repeated once daily for 5–10 days postoperatively. **In malignancy:** 2,500 international units 1–2 hr before surgery followed by 2,500 international units 12 hr later and 5,000 international units once daily for 5–10 days postoperatively.

*Prevention of DVT following hip replacement surgery.*

**Adults:** 2,500 international units within 2 hr before surgery with a second dose of 2,500 international units in the evening on the day of surgery (6 or more hr after the first dose). If surgery occurs in the evening, omit the second dose on the day of surgery. On the first postoperative day, give 5,000 international units once daily for 5–10 days. Alternatively, can give 5,000 international units the evening before surgery, followed by 5,000 international units once daily for 5–10 days, starting the evening of the day of surgery.

*Severely restricted mobility during acute illness.*

**Adults:** Give 5,000 international units once daily for up to 12 to 14 days.

*Prevent ischemic complications in unstable angina/non-Q-wave MI.*

**Adults:** 120 international units/kg, not to exceed 10,000 international units q 12 hr with concurrent PO aspirin (75–165 mg/day). Continue treatment until client is clinically stabilized (usually 5–8 days).

*Venous thromboembolism in clients with cancer.*

**Adults, first 30 days of treatment:** 200 units/kg total body weight once daily, not to exceed 18,000 units per day.
**Months 2–6:** Approximately 150 units/kg once daily, not to exceed 18,000 units per day. Safety and efficacy beyond 6 months have not been determined.

*Thrombocytopenia in clients with cancer and acute symptomatic venous thromboembolism.*

**Adults: Platelet counts between 50,000 and 100,000/mm³:** Reduce the daily dose by 2,500 units until platelet count recovers to at least 100,000/mm³. **Platelets less than 50,000/ mm³:** Discontinue dalteparin until platelet count recovers above 50,000/mm³.

**NEED TO KNOW**

1. When neuraxial anesthesia (spinal/epidural anesthesia) or spinal puncture is used, those who are anticoagulated or scheduled to be anticoagulated with low molecular weight heparins or heparinoids for prevention of thromboembolic complications are at risk of developing a spinal or epidural hematoma that can result in long-term or permanent paralysis.
2. Do not mix with other infusions or injections unless compatibility data known.
3. Give by deep SC injection while sitting or lying down. May give in a U-shape area around the navel, the upper outer side of the thigh, or the upper outer quadrangle of the buttock. Change/rotate the injection site daily.
4. Avoid OTC aspirin containing products. Use electric razor and soft toothbrush to prevent tissue trauma.
5. Report any unusual bruising/bleeding or hemorrhage. Therapy may last for 5–10 days.

# Diazepam

(dye-**AYZ**-eh-pam)

**Rx:** Diastat AcuDial, Diazepam Intensol, Valium, **C-IV.**

**CLASSIFICATION(S):** Antianxiety drug, benzodiazepine

**USES: PO:** (1) Management of anxiety disorders or for short-term relief of symptoms of anxiety. (2) Adjunct for relief of skeletal muscle spasm caused by reflex spasm to local pathology (e.g., inflammation of muscles or joints or secondary to trauma). Also, spasticity due to upper motor neuron disorders (e.g., cerebral palsy, paraplegia). Athetosis, stiff-man syndrome. (3) Acute alcohol withdrawal for symptomatic relief of acute agitation, tremor, impending or acute delirum tremens, and hallucinosis. **Parenteral:** (1) Adjunct therapy in status epilepticus and severe recurrent convulsive seizures. (2) IV prior to cardioversion for relief of anxiety and tension and to decrease client's recall. (3) Relief of anxiety and tension in those undergoing surgical procedures. As an adjunct prior to endoscopic or surgical procedures if apprehension, anxiety, or acute stress reactions are present; also, to diminish client recall of the procedures. (4) Adjunct for the relief of skeletal muscle spasm due to reflex spasm caused by local pathology (e.g., inflammation of muscles or joints, secondary to trauma). Also, spasticity due to upper motor neuron disorders (e.g., cerebral palsy, paraplegia); athetosis; stiff-man syndrome. (5) Symptomatic relief of acute agitation, tremor, impending or acute delirium tremens, and hallucinosis. **Rectal gel:** Management of selective refractory clients with epilepsy who are stable on regimens of anticonvulsant drugs who require intermittent diazepam to control increased seizure activity.

**ACTION/KINETICS:** Reduces anxiety by increasing or facilitating the inhibitory neurotransmitter activity of GABA. The skeletal muscle relaxant effect may be due to enhancement of GABA-mediated presynaptic inhibition at the spinal level as well as in the brain stem reticular formation. **Onset: PO,** 30–60 min; **IM,** 15–30 min; **IV,** more rapid. **Peak plasma levels: PO,** 0.5–2 hr; **IM,** 0.5–1.5; **IV,** 0.25 hr. **Duration:** 3 hr. **t½:** 20–50 hr. Metabolized in the liver to the active metabolites. Diazepam and metabolites are excreted through the urine.

**SIDE EFFECTS:** Drowsiness (transient), ataxia, confusion.

---

**DOSAGE: Oral Solution; Solution, Intensol; Tablets**

*Management and relief of anxiety disorders.*

**Adults:** 2–10 mg 2 to 4 times per day. **Elderly clients or in presence of debilitating disease, initial:** 2–2.5 mg 1 or 2 times per day; **then,** increase gradually as needed and tolerated.

*Acute alcohol withdrawal.*

**Adults:** 10 mg 3 or 4 times per day during the first 24 hr; reduce to 5 mg 3 or 4 times per day, as needed.

*Adjunct in skeletal muscle spasms.*

**Adults:** 2–10 mg 3 or 4 times per day.

*Adjunct in convulsive disorders.*

**Adults:** 2–10 mg 2–4 times per day. **Elderly or debilitated clients, initial:** 2–2.5 mg 1 or 2 times per day; **then,** increase dose gradually as needed and tolerated. Limit dose to the smallest effective amount to preclude development of ataxia or oversedation.

**DOSAGE: IM; IV**

*Moderate anxiety disorders and symptoms of anxiety.*

**Adults:** 2–5 mg IM or IV. Repeat in 3–4 hr if needed.

*Severe anxiety disorders and symptoms of anxiety.*

**Adults:** 5–10 mg IM or IV. Repeat in 3–4 hr if needed.

*Acute alcohol withdrawal.*

**Adults, initial:** 10 mg IM or IV; **then,** 5–10 mg in 3–4 hr if needed.

*Endoscopic procedures.*

**Adults, IV:** Titrate dosage to desired sedative response (e.g., slurring of speech). Give slowly and just prior to procedure. Reduce narcotic dosage by at least one-third; in some cases, narcotics may be omitted. **Usual:** 10 mg or less; up to 20 mg may be used, especially when concomitant narcotics are omitted. **IM:** 5–10 mg 30 min prior to procedure if IV route cannot be used.

*Muscle spasms.*
**Adults, initial:** 5–10 mg IM or IV; **then,** 5–10 mg in 3–4 hr if needed. Tetanus may require larger doses.

*Preoperative medication.*
**Adults:** 10 mg IM before surgery. If atropine, scopolamine, or other premedications are desired, use separate syringes.

*Cardioversion.*
**Adults:** 5–15 mg IV, 5–10 min prior to procedure.

*Status epilepticus or severe recurrent convulsive seizures.*
**Adults, initial:** 5–10 mg IV (preferred); **then,** may be repeated at 10–15 min intervals up to a maximum of 30 mg, if needed. May repeat therapy in 2–4 hr. Use with extreme caution in chronic lung disease or unstable cardiovascular status.

**DOSAGE: Rectal Gel**
**Adults:** Depending on age dose ranges from 0.2–0.5 mg/kg; calculate the recommended dose by rounding up to the next available unit dose. If needed, a second dose may be given 4–12 hr after the first dose. Do not treat more than 5 episodes/month or more than 1 episode q 5 days. **Adults:** 0.2 mg/kg. In the elderly or debilitated, adjust dose downward to reduce ataxia or oversedation.

**NEED TO KNOW**
1. When used as an adjunct for seizure disorders, diazepam may increase the frequency or severity of clonic-tonic seizures, for which an increase in the dose of anticonvulsant medication is necessary.
2. Use IV diazepam with extreme caution in the elderly, in very ill clients, and in those with limited pulmonary reserve as apnea or cardiac arrest may occur.
3. Mix Intensol solution with beverages such as water, soda, and

juices or soft foods such as applesauce or puddings. Use only the calibrated dropper provided to withdraw drug; once withdrawn and mixed, use immediately.

4. The rectal delivery system includes a plastic applicator with a flexible, molded tip available in two lengths. The Diastat AcuDial 2.5 mg and 10 mg syringes are available with a 4.4 cm tip and the Diastat AcuDial 20 mg syringe is available with a 6 cm tip.

5. IV diazepam will control seizures promptly; however, many clients experience a return to seizure activity (probably due to the short duration of IV diazepam). Be prepared to readminister.

6. Diazepam is not recommended for maintenance of seizure control. Consider other agents for long-term control.

7. Parenteral administration may cause bradycardia, respiratory/cardiac arrest; have emergency equipment/drugs available.

8. Due to the possibility of precipitation and instability, do not infuse diazepam. Do not mix or dilute with other solutions or drugs in the syringe or infusion container.

9. May cause dizziness/drowsiness; avoid activities that require mental alertness until drug effects realized.

10. Smoking may increase drug metabolism, thus requiring higher dose than nonsmoker. Do not stop drug abruptly.

## Diclofenac epolamine
(dye-**KLOH**-fen-ack)

**Rx:** Flector.

## Diclofenac potassium

**Rx:** Cataflam.

## Diclofenac sodium

**Rx: Gel:** Solaraze. **Ophthalmic:** Voltaren. **Tablets:** Voltaren, Voltaren-XR.

**CLASSIFICATION(S):** Nonsteroidal anti-inflammatory

**USES: PO, Immediate-release (Diclofenac potassium):** (1) Acute and chronic treatment of signs and symptoms of rheumatoid arthritis and osteoarthritis. (2) Ankylosing spondylitis. (3) Mild-to-moderate pain. (4) Use immediate-release when prompt relief is desired. **PO, Delayed-Release or Extended-Release (Diclofenac sodium):** (1) Signs and symptoms of rheumatoid arthritis and osteoarthritis. (2) Acute or long-term use for ankylosing spondylitis (delayed-release). **Transdermal Patch (Diclofenac epolamine):** Topical treatment of acute pain due to minor strains, sprains, and contusions. **Ophthalmic:** (1) Postoperative inflammation following cataract removal. (2) Temporary relief of pain and photophobia following corneal refractive surgery.

**ACTION/KINETICS:** Anti-inflammatory effect is due to inhibition of the enzyme cyclo-oxygenase. Inhibition of cyclo-oxygenase results in decreased prostaglandin synthesis. Prostaglandin will cause inflammation. Effective in reducing joint swelling, pain, and morning stiffness and increases mobility in those with inflammatory disease. *Immediate-release product:* **Onset:** 30 min. **Peak plasma levels:** 1 hr. **Duration:** 8 hr. *Delayed-release product:* **Peak plasma levels:** 2–3 hr. **t½:** 1–2 hr. For all dosage forms, food will affect the rate, but not the amount, absorbed from the GI tract. Metabolized in the liver and excreted by the kidneys.

**SIDE EFFECTS: After PO use:** Headache, dizzness, abdominal pain/cramps, nausea, diarrhea, constipation, dyspepsia/indigestion.

**DOSAGE: Tablets, Immediate-Release** Diclofenac potassium

*Analgesia.*
   **Adults, initial:** 50 mg 3 times per day of immediate-release tablets. In some, an initial dose of 100 mg followed by 50-mg doses may achieve better results. After the first day, the total daily dose should not exceed 150 mg.

*Rheumatoid arthritis.*
   **Adults:** 150–200 mg/day in divided doses (e.g., 50 mg 3 or 4 times per day). Do not exceed 225 mg/day.

*Osteoarthritis.*
   **Adults:** 100–150 mg/day in divided doses (e.g., 50 mg 2 or 3 times per day). Doses greater than 200 mg/day have not been evaluated.

*Ankylosing spondylitis.*
   **Adults:** 50 mg 2 times per day; **range:** 100–125 mg/day. Doses greater than 125 mg/day have not been evaluated.

**DOSAGE: Delayed-Release Tablets** Diclofenac sodium

*Ankylosing spondylitis.*
   **Adults:** 100–125 mg/day, given as 25 mg 4 times per day, with an extra 25 mg at bedtime, if necessary.

*Osteoarthritis.*
   **Adults:** 100–150 mg/day (e.g., 50 mg 2 or 3 times per day or 75 mg 2 times per day).

*Rheumatoid arthritis.*
   **Adults:** 150–200 mg/day in divided doses (50 mg 3 or 4 times per day or 75 mg 2 times per day).

**DOSAGE: Extended-Release Tablets**

*Osteoarthritis.*
   **Adults:** 100 mg/day.

*Rheumatoid arthritis.*
   **Adults:** 100 mg/day. If this dose is not satisfactory, dose may

be increased to 100 mg 2 times per day if the benefits out-weigh the risk of increased side effects.

**DOSAGE: Ophthalmic Solution, 0.1%**

*Following cataract surgery.*

**Adults:** 1 gtt in the affected eye 4 times per day beginning 24 hr after cataract surgery and for 2 weeks thereafter.

*Corneal refractive surgery.*

**Adults:** 1–2 gtt within 1 hr prior to surgery; then, apply 1–2 gtt within 15 min of surgery and continue 4 times per day for up to 3 days.

**DOSAGE: Transdermal Patch**

*Acute pain due to minor strains, sprains, contusions.*

**Adults:** Apply 1 patch to the most painful area twice a day. Change patch once every 12 hr. Remove patch if irritation occurs.

**NEED TO KNOW**

1. NSAIDs may cause an increased risk of serious CV thrombotic events, MI, and stroke, which can be fatal.
2. NSAIDs cause an increased risk of serious GI side effects including inflammation, bleeding, ulceration, and perforation of the stomach or intestines, which can be fatal.
3. Do not use to treat perioperative pain following coronary artery bypass graft surgery.
4. In those weighing less than 60 kg (132 lbs) or where the severity of the disease, concomitant medications, or other diseases warrant, reduce the maximum recommended total dose of diclofenac potassium.
5. The various dosage forms are not necessarily bioequivalent even if the milligram strength is the same.
6. Take with meals, a full glass of water or milk if GI upset occurs; remain upright for 30 min after taking drug to reduce esophageal irritation.
7. Clients with diabetes should monitor blood sugar levels closely; may alter response to antidiabetic agents.

8. Report adverse effects, changes in stools, ringing in ears, stomach pain, unusual bruising/bleeding, lack of response.

## Digoxin A
(dih-**JOX**-in)
**Rx:** Digitek, Lanoxicaps, Lanoxin.

**CLASSIFICATION(S):** Cardiac glycoside

**USES:** (1) CHF, including that due to venous congestion, edema, dyspnea, orthopnea, and cardiac arrhythmia. May be drug of choice for CHF because of rapid onset, relatively short duration, and ability to be administered PO or IV. (2) Control of rapid ventricular contraction rate in clients with atrial fibrillation or flutter. (3) Slow HR in sinus tachycardia due to CHF. (4) SVT. (5) Prophylaxis and treatment of recurrent paroxysmal atrial tachycardia with paroxysmal AV junctional rhythm. (6) Cardiogenic shock (value not established).

**ACTION/KINETICS:** Increases the force and velocity of myocardial contraction (positive inotropic effect). This effect is due to inhibition of sodium/potassium–ATPase in the sarcolemmal membrane, which alters excitation-contraction coupling. Inhibiting sodium/potassium–ATPase results in increased calcium influx and increased release of free calcium ions within the myocardial cells, which then potentiate the contractility of cardiac muscle fibers. Digoxin also decreases HR, decreases the rate of conduction, and increases the refractory period of the AV node due to an increase in parasympathetic tone and a decrease in sympathetic tone. **Onset: PO:** 0.5–2 hr; **time to peak effect:** 2–6 hr. **Duration:** Over 24 hr. **Onset, IV:** 5–30 min; **time to peak effect:** 1–4 hr. **Duration:** 6 days. **t½:** 30–40 hr. **Therapeutic serum level:** 0.5–2.0 ng/mL. Serum levels above 2.5 ng/mL indicate toxicity. Fifty percent to 70% is excreted unchanged by the kidneys.

**SIDE EFFECTS:** Tachycardia, headache, dizziness, mental disturbances, N&V, diarrhea, anorexia, blurred or yellow vision.

Digoxin is extremely toxic and has caused **death** even in clients who have received the drug for long periods of time. There is a narrow margin of safety between an effective therapeutic dose and a toxic dose. *DEATH MOST OFTEN RESULTS FROM VENTRICULAR FIBRILLATION.*

## DOSAGE: Capsules

*Digitalization: Rapid.*

**Adults:** 0.4–0.6 mg initially followed by 0.1–0.3 mg q 6–8 hr until desired effect achieved.

*Digitalization: Slow.*

**Adults:** A total of 0.05–0.35 mg/day divided in two doses for a period of 7–22 days to reach steady-state serum levels.

*Maintenance.*

**Adults:** 0.05–0.35 mg once or twice daily.

## DOSAGE: Elixir; Tablets

*Digitalization: Rapid.*

**Adults:** A total of 0.75–1.25 mg divided into two or more doses each given at 6–8-hr intervals.

*Digitalization: Slow.*

**Adults:** 0.125–0.5 mg/day for 7 days.

*Maintenance.*

**Adults:** 0.125–0.5 mg/day.

## DOSAGE: IV

*Digitalization.*

**Adults:** Same as tablets. **Maintenance:** 0.125–0.5 mg/day in divided doses or as a single dose.

## NEED TO KNOW

1. Use with caution in clients with ischemic heart disease, acute myocarditis, hypertrophic subaortic stenosis, hypoxic or myxedemic states, Adams-Stokes or carotid sinus syndromes, cardiac amyloidosis, or cyanotic heart and lung disease, including emphysema and partial heart block.

2. Electric pacemakers may sensitize the myocardium to cardiac glycosides.
3. Use with caution and at reduced dosage in elderly, debilitated clients. The half-life of digoxin is prolonged in the elderly.
4. Measure liquids precisely using calibrated dropper/syringe.
5. Differences in bioavailability have been noted between products; monitor when changing from one product to another.
6. For clients being digitalized and for clients on maintenance dose digoxin: (a) With digitalization, monitor closely. (b) Observe and monitor for bradycardia/arrhythmias; count apical rate for at least 1 min before administering drug.
7. If taking non-potassium-sparing diuretics as well as digoxin, will need potassium supplements.
8. If gastric distress experienced, use antacid. Antacids containing Al or Mg and kaolin/pectin mixtures should be given 6 hr before or 6 hr after dose of cardiac glycoside to prevent decreased therapeutic effects.
9. Take after meals to lessen gastric irritation.
10. Do not take with grapefruit juice.
11. Follow directions carefully for taking medication. If one dose is accidentally missed, do not double up on the next dose.
12. Report adverse effects or toxic drug symptoms: Anorexia, N&V, abdominal pain, and diarrhea are often early symptoms due to the toxic effects on the GI tract and chemoreceptor trigger zone stimulation. Disorientation, agitation, visual disturbances, changes in color perception, irregular heartbeat, and hallucinations may also occur.
13. Report persistent cough, difficulty breathing, or swelling (S&S of CHF).

# Diltiazem hydrochloride
(dill-**TIE**-ah-zem)

**C**

**Rx: Capsule, Extended-Release:** Cardizem CD, Cartia XT, Dilacor XR, Dilt-CD, Dilt-XR, Diltia XT, Diltiazem HCl Extended Release, Taztia XT, Tiazac. **Injection:** Cardizem. **Tablets, Extended-Release:** Cardizem LA. **Tablets, Immediate-Release:** Cardizem.

**CLASSIFICATION(S):** Calcium channel blocker

**USES: PO:** (1) Angina pectoris due to coronary artery spasm. (2) Chronic stable angina (classic effort-associated angina). (3) Hypertension (extended- or sustained-release only). **Parenteral:** (1) Temporary control of rapid ventricular rate in atrial fibrillation or flutter. (2) Rapid conversion of paroxysmal SVT to sinus rhythm.

**ACTION/KINETICS:** Inhibits influx of calcium through the cell membrane, resulting in a depression of automaticity and conduction velocity in cardiac muscle. Decreases SA and AV conduction and prolongs AV node effective and functional refractory periods. Also decreases myocardial contractility and peripheral vascular resistance. Slight decrease in HR. **Tablets, Immediate-Release: Onset,** 30–60 min; **time to peak plasma levels:** 2–4 hr; $t^1/_2$, **elimination:** about 3–4.5 hr (5–8 hr with high and repetitive doses); **duration:** 4–8 hr. **Extended-Release Capsules/Tablets: Onset,** 2–3 hr; **time to peak plasma levels:** 10–14 hr; $t^1/_2$, **elimination:** 4–9.5 hr; **duration:** 12 hr. **IV, $t^1/_2$, elimination:** About 3.4 hr. **Therapeutic serum levels:** 0.05–0.2 mcg/mL. Metabolized in the liver to desacetyldiltiazem, which manifests 25–50% of the activity of diltiazem. Excreted through both the bile and urine.

**SIDE EFFECTS:** AV block, bradycardia, edema, dizziness/lightheadedness, headache, pain, dyspnea, rhinitis, infection. *ARRHYTHMIAS, ABNORMAL ECG, VENTRICULAR EXTRASYSTOLES, STEVENS-JOHNSON SYNDROME, BUNDLE BRANCH BLOCK.*

**DOSAGE: Tablets, Immediate-Release**

*Angina.*

**Adults, initial:** Individualize dose. 30 mg 4 times per day before meals and at bedtime; **then,** increase gradually to total daily dose of 180–360 mg (given in three to four divided doses). Increments may be made q 1–2 days until the optimum response is attained.

**DOSAGE: Tablets, Extended-Release**

*Hypertension.*

**Adults, initial, monotherapy:** Individualize dose. 180–240 mg once daily; some may respond to lower doses. May be titrated to a maximum dose of 540 mg/day. Schedule dosage adjustments accordingly as maximum effect usually seen within 14 days.

*Angina.*

**Adults, initial:** Individualize dose. 180 mg; **then,** may increase dose at intervals of 7–14 days if adequate response not obtained. Doses above 360 mg appear not to have any additional benefit.

**DOSAGE: Capsules, Extended-Release**

*Angina.*

**Adults: Cardizem CD and Cartia XT: Initial,** 120 or 180 mg once daily. Up to 480 mg/day may be required. Dosage adjustments should be carried out over a 7–14-day period. **Dilacor XR and Diltia XT: Initial,** 120 mg once daily; **then,** dose may be titrated, depending on the needs of the client, up to 480 mg once daily. Titration may be carried out over a 7–14-day period. **Tiazac: Initial,** 120–180 once daily. Some may respond to higher doses up to 540 mg once daily. When necessary, carry out titration over 7–14 days.

*Hypertension.*

**Adults: Cardizem CD and Cartia XT: Initial,** 180–240 mg once daily. Some respond to lower doses. Maximum antihypertensive effect usually reached within 14 days. Usual range is 240–360 mg once daily. **Dilacor XR and Diltia XT: Initial,** 180–240 mg once daily. Clients 60 years and older may respond to a lower dose of 120 mg. Usual range is 180–480 mg once daily. The dose may be increased to 540 mg/day with little or no increased risk of side effects. May be used alone or in combination with other antihypertensive drugs, such as diuretics. **Tiazac: Initial,** 120–240 mg once daily. Maximum effect usually reached by 14 days of therapy; thus, schedule dosage adjustments accordingly. Usual range is 120–540 mg once daily. May be used alone or with other antihypertensive drugs.

## DOSAGE: IV Bolus

*Atrial fibrillation/flutter; paroxysmal SVT.*

**Adults, initial:** 0.25 mg/kg (average 20 mg) given over 2 min; **then,** if response is inadequate, a second dose may be given after 15 min. The second bolus dose is 0.35 mg/kg (average 25 mg) given over 2 min. Subsequent doses should be individualized. Some clients may respond to an initial dose of 0.15 mg/kg (duration of action may be shorter).

## DOSAGE: IV, Continuous Infusion

*Atrial fibrillation/flutter.*

**Adults, initial:** For continuous reduction of HR (up to 24 hr) for those with atrial fibrillation/flutter, begin an IV infusion immediately after the IV bolus dose. Initial infusion rate is 10 mg/hr; may be increased in 5 mg increments to 15 mg/hr. Infusion longer than 24 hr at a dose of 15 mg/hr is not recommended.

---

### NEED TO KNOW

1. Do not use in hypotension, cardiogenic shock, second- or third-degree AV block, or sick sinus syndrome except in presence of a functioning ventricular pacemaker.
2. The half-life may be increased in geriatric clients. Use with caution in hepatic disease and in CHF.
3. Use with beta blockers or digitalis is usually well tolerated, but the combined effects cannot be predicted, especially with cardiac conduction abnormalities or LV dysfunction.

4. Do not give diltiazem injection, Cardizem LyoJect, and Cardizem Monovial in the same IV line.
5. Take extended-release capsules on an empty stomach. Do not open, chew, or crush; swallow whole.
6. Use caution; may cause drowsiness/dizziness.
7. Rise slowly from a lying to a sitting and standing position; may cause a drop in BP.
8. Report persistent/bothersome side effects including headaches, constipation, unusual tiredness, or weakness.
9. Continue carrying short-acting nitrites (nitroglycerin) at all times; use as directed.

---

**Docusate calcium (Dioctyl calcium sulfosuccinate)** **C**
(**DOCK**-you-sayt)
**OTC:** DC Softgels, Pro-Cal-Sof, Sulfolax Calcium, Surfak Liquigels.
**Docusate sodium (Dioctyl sodium sulfosuccinate)**
**OTC:** Colace, D-S-S, D.O.S., Dioctyn Softgels, Docu, Dulcolax Stool Softener, Ex-Lax Stool Softener, Gena Soft, Non-Habit Forming Stool Softener, Phillips Liqui-Gels, Regulex SS, Silace Stool Softener, Sof-lax.

**CLASSIFICATION(S):** Laxative, emollient
**USES:** (1) To lessen strain of defecation in persons with hernia or CV diseases or other diseases in which straining at stool should be avoided. (2) Megacolon or bedridden clients. (3) Constipation associated with dry, hard stools.
**ACTION/KINETICS:** Acts by lowering the surface tension of the feces and promoting penetration by water and fat, thus increasing the softness of the fecal mass. Does not seem to interfere with the absorption of nutrients. **Onset:** 12–72 hr.
**SIDE EFFECTS:** Diarrhea, N&V, perianal irritation, flatulence, cramps.

**DOSAGE: Capsules** DOCUSATE CALCIUM

*Laxative.*

**Adults:** 240 mg/day until bowel movements are normal.

**DOSAGE: Capsules; Capsules; Soft Gel; Oral Liquid; Syrup; Tablets** DOCUSATE SODIUM

*Laxative.*

**Adults:** 50–500 mg, depending on the product.

**NEED TO KNOW**

1. May give oral solutions with milk or juices to help mask bitter taste.
2. Drink a glass of water with each dose.
3. Because docusate salts are minimally absorbed, it may require 1–3 days to soften fecal matter.

---

## Donepezil hydrochloride
(dohn-**EP**-eh-zil)                                            **C**

**Rx:** Aricept, Aricept ODT.

**CLASSIFICATION(S):** Treatment of Alzheimer's disease
**USES:** Treatment of mild to severe dementia of the Alzheimer's type. Is combined with memantine (Namenda) to lower the decline of mental and physical function in Alzheimer's disease.
**ACTION/KINETICS:** Donepezil, a cholinesterase inhibitor, exerts its effect by enhancing cholinergic function by increasing levels of acetylcholine through reversible inhibition of acetylcholinesterase. No evidence that the drug alters the course of the underlying dementing process. Well absorbed from the GI tract. **Peak plasma levels:** 3–4 hr; steady state reached in 15 days. Food does not affect the rate or extent of absorption. **t½, elimination:** 70 hr. Metabolized in the liver, and both unchanged drug and metabolites are excreted in the urine and feces.
**SIDE EFFECTS:** Anorexia, diarrhea, fatigue, insomnia, muscle

cramps, N&V, dizziness, headache, ecchymosis. *SEIZURES, HEMORRHAGE, HEART FAILURE.*

## DOSAGE: Oral Solution; Tablets; Tablets, Oral Disintegrating

*Mild to moderate Alzheimer's disease.*

**Adults, initial:** 5 or 10 mg once daily. Use of a 10-mg dose did not provide a clinical effect greater than the 5-mg dose; however, in some clients, 10 mg daily may be superior. Do not increase the dose to 10 mg until clients have been on a daily dose of 5 mg for 4 to 6 weeks.

*Severe Alzheimer's disease.*

**Adults:** 10 mg given once daily. Do not achieve a dose of 10 mg until clients have been on a daily dose of 5 mg for 4–6 weeks.

### NEED TO KNOW

1. Use with caution in clients with a history of asthma or obstructive pulmonary disease.
2. Take in the evening, just prior to bedtime. May take with or without food.
3. Place the oral disintegrating tablet on the tongue; after the tablet dissolves, drink water.
4. Report adverse effects including irregular pulse or dizzy spells, lack of response, worsening of symptoms.

## Duloxetine hydrochloride     **C**
(doo-**LOX**-eh-teen)
**Rx:** Cymbalta.

**CLASSIFICATION(S):** Antidepressant, selective serotonin and norepinephrine reuptake inhibitor
**USES:** (1) Treatment of major depressive disorder as defined in the DSM-IV. (2) Management of neuropathic pain associated with

diabetic peripheral neuropathy. (3) Treatment of generalized anxiety disorder.

**ACTION/KINETICS:** Antidepressant and pain inhibitory effect believed to be related to potentiation of serotonergic and noradrenergic activity in the CNS. Well absorbed after PO administration. **Maximum plasma levels:** 6 hr (there is a 2-hr lag until absorption begins). Food delays the time to peak levels from 6 to 10 hr. There is a 3-hr delay in absorption and a one-third increase in apparent clearance after an evening dose compared with a morning dose. Undergoes extensive metabolism by the liver isoenzymes, CYP2D6 and CYP1A2. $t\frac{1}{2}$, **elimination:** 8–17 hr. Excreted in both the urine (70%) and feces (20%).

**SIDE EFFECTS:** N&V, somnolence, dizziness, headache, constipation, dry mouth, fatigue, insomnia, decreased appetite, increased sweating. *COMPLETED SUICIDE, SEIZURES.*

---

**DOSAGE: Capsules, Delayed-Release**

*Major depressive disorder.*

**Adults, initial:** 20 mg twice a day to 60 mg/day (given either once a day or 30 mg twice a day) without regard to meals. There is no evidence that doses greater than 60 mg/day confer additional benefits. Periodically evaluate to determine need for maintenance treatment.

*Diabetic peripheral neuropathic pain.*

**Adults, initial:** 60 mg/day given once a day without regard to meals. Periodically evaluate to determine need for maintenance treatment; efficacy beyond 12 weeks has not been evaluated.

*Generalized anxiety disorder.*

**Adults, initial:** 60 mg once daily without regard to meals. For some, it may be beneficial to start at 30 mg once daily for 1 week to allow adjustment to the drug before increasing to 60 mg once daily. Efficacy of duloxetine for more than 10 weeks has not been evaluated. Periodically evaluate the long-term usefulness of the drug.

## NEED TO KNOW

1. Do not use in end-stage renal disease or severe renal impairment ($C_{CR}$ less than 30 mL/min), any hepatic insufficiency, chronic liver disease, substantial alcohol use, uncontrolled narrow-angle glaucoma, or concomitant use in those taking MAOIs.

2. Adults with major depressive disorder may experience worsening of their depression and/or suicidal ideation and behavior, whether or not they are taking antidepressant medication.

3. Use with caution in clients with a history of mania, seizure disorder, with controlled narrow-angle glaucoma, in the elderly, and with conditions that may slow gastric emptying.

4. Treatment for several months or longer may be needed for acute episodes of major depression. Periodically reassess clients to determine need for and appropriate dose for maintenance therapy.

5. Abrupt discontinuation may cause dizziness, N&V, headache, paresthesia, irritability, and nightmares. Reduce dose gradually rather than abruptly discontinuing the drug.

6. Wait at least 14 days between discontinuing a MAOI and initiating duloxetine. Also, at least 5 days should elapse after stopping duloxetine and starting a MAOI.

7. Do not chew, crush, or sprinkle contents, or mix with liquids; swallow whole to protect enteric coating.

8. May experience dizziness, N&V, headache, paresthesia, irritability, and nightmares. Do not stop suddenly; reduce dose gradually. Report adverse new onset side effects, especially worsening of depression, inability to sleep, suicide thoughts, anxiety, agitation, hostility, and impulsiveness.

9. Avoid heavy alcohol use; may cause severe liver injury.

**CLASSIFICATION(S):** Antiparkinson drug

**USES:** As an adjunct with levodopa/carbidopa to treat idiopathic parkinsonism clients who experience signs and symptoms of end-of-dose 'wearing off.'

**ACTION/KINETICS:** A selective and reversible catechol-O-methyltransferase (COMT) inhibitor. COMT eliminates catechols (e.g., dopa, dopamine, norepinephrine, epinephrine) and in the presence of a decarboxylase inhibitor (e.g., carbidopa), COMT becomes the major metabolizing enzyme for dopa. Thus, in the presence of a COMT inhibitor, levels of dopa and dopamine increase. When entacapone is given with levodopa and carbidopa, plasma levels of levodopa are greater and more sustained than after levodopa/carbidopa alone. This leads to more constant dopaminergic stimulation in the brain resulting in improvement of the signs and symptoms of Parkinson's disease. Rapidly absorbed. Almost completely metabolized in the liver with most excreted in the feces. $t\frac{1}{2}$, **elimination:** Biphasic 0.4–0.7 hr and 2.4 hr.

**SIDE EFFECTS:** Dyskinesia, nausea, hyperkinesia, diarrhea, urine discoloration, hypokinesia, dizziness, abdominal pain, constipation, fatigue.

---

**DOSAGE: Tablets**

*Parkinsonism.*

**Adults:** 200 mg given concomitantly with each levodopa/carbidopa dose up to a maximum of 8 times per day (i.e., 1,600 mg/day).

---

**NEED TO KNOW**

1. Use with caution with drugs known to be metabolized by COMT (e.g., apomorphine, bitolterol, dobutamine, dopamine, epinephrine, isoetharine, isoproterenol, methyldopa, norepi-

nephrine) due to the possibility of increased HR, arrhythmias, and excessive changes in BP.

2. Always give in combination with levodopa/carbidopa; entacapone has no antiparkinson effect by itself.

3. Most clients required a decreased daily levodopa dose (about 25%) if their daily levodopa dose was 800 mg or more, or if they had moderate or severe dyskinesias prior to entacapone treatment.

4. Rapid withdrawal or abrupt reduction in entacapone dose can lead to emergence of S&S of parkinsonism and could lead to a complex resembling neuroleptic malignant syndrome (hyperpyrexia and confusion).

5. Take as directed with levodopa/carbidopa with or without food. Do not crush or chew tablets.

6. May experience loss of consciousness, nausea, diarrhea, hallucinations, increase in involuntary movements, altered pulmonary or kidney function. Report if evident.

7. Urine may appear brownish-orange in color.

8. Rise slowly from a sitting or lying position to prevent sudden drop in BP or dizziness.

---

### Epoetin alfa recombinant
(ee-**POH**-ee-tin)
**Rx:** Epogen, Procrit.

**CLASSIFICATION(S):** Erythropoietin, human recombinant
**USES:** (1) Treatment of anemia associated with chronic renal failure in adults, including clients on dialysis (end-stage renal disease) or adults not on dialysis. (2) Zidovudine-induced anemia in HIV-infected clients to decrease the need for transfusions. (3) Treatment of anemia in clients with nonmyeloid malignancies in which anemia is due to the effect of coadministered chemotherapy. (4) Treatment of anemic clients (hemoglobin more than 10 to less than 13 grams/dL) to reduce allogeneic blood transfusions in

clients scheduled to undergo elective, noncardiac, nonvascular surgery.

**ACTION/KINETICS:** Has the identical amino acid sequence and same biologic effects as endogenous erythropoietin (which is normally synthesized in the kidney and stimulates RBC production). Epoetin alfa will stimulate RBC production and thus elevate or maintain the RBC level, decreasing the need for blood transfusions. **t½:** 4–13 hr in clients with chronic renal failure, but is about 20% longer in those with chronic renal failure compared with healthy subjects. **Peak serum levels after SC:** 5–24 hr.

**SIDE EFFECTS:** Hypertension, headache, fatigue, N&V, diarrhea, edema, asthenia, respiratory congestion, cough, pyrexia, rash, SOB, insomnia, pruritus, DVT (in surgery clients). *MI, SEIZURES, ANAPHYLAXIS*.

---

**DOSAGE: IV; SC**

*Chronic renal failure.*

**Adults, IV, initial (dialysis or nondialysis clients), SC (nondialysis clients):** 50–100 units/kg 3 times per week. The rate of increase of hematocrit depends on both dosage and client variation. **Maintenance, nondialysis clients:** Individualize; 75–150 units/kg week have maintained hematocrits of 36–38% for up to 6 months; **hemodialysis clients:** 12.5–525 units/kg 3 times per week (median dose is 75 units/kg 3 times per week). **Maintenance, peritoneal dialysis clients:** 24–323 units/kg/week given in divided doses 2–3 times per week. Median dosage is 76 units/kg/week in divided doses.

*NOTE:* Reduce dose by about 25% if hemoglobin approaches 12 grams/dL or if hemoglobin increases by more than 1 gram/dL in any 2-week period. Increase dose if hemoglobin does not increase by 2 grams/dL after 8 weeks of therapy and hemoglobin remains at a level not sufficient to avoid the need for RBC transfusion.

*Zidovudine-treated, HIV infections.*

**Adults, initial, IV, SC:** 100 units/kg 3 times per week for 8 weeks (in clients with serum erythropoietin levels less than or equal to 500 milliunits/mL who are receiving less than or equal to 4,200 mg/week of zidovudine). If a satisfactory response is obtained, the dose can be increased by 50–100 units/kg 3 times per week. Evaluate the response q 4–8 weeks thereafter with dosage adjusted by 50–100 units/kg increments 3 times per week. If clients have not responded to 300 units/kg 3 times per week, it is not likely they will respond to higher doses. If the hemoglobin exceeds 12 grams/dL, discontinue the dose until the hemoglobin drops below 11 grams/dL. Reduce the dose by 25% when treatment is resumed and then titrate to maintain the desired hemoglobin.

*Cancer clients on chemotherapy.*
**Adults, initial, SC:** 150 units/kg three times per week.

*Surgery to reduce allogeneic blood transfusions.*
**Adults, SC:** 300 units/kg/day for 10 days before surgery, on the day of surgery, and for 4 days after surgery. Alternative: 600 units/kg SC once a week 21, 14, and 7 days before surgery plus a fourth dose on the day of surgery. Iron supplementation is required at the time of epoetin therapy and continuing throughout the course of therapy.

## NEED TO KNOW

1. Use the lowest dose of epoetin alfa that will gradually increase the hemoglobin concentration to the lowest level sufficient to avoid the need for red blood cell transfusion.
2. Epoetin alfa and other erythropoiesis-stimulating agents increased the risk of death and serious CV reactions when administered to target a hemoglobin of more than 12 grams/dL.
3. Do not use in chronic renal failure clients who need severe anemia corrected or to treat anemia in HIV-infected or cancer clients due to factors such as iron or folate deficiencies, hemolysis, or GI bleeding.
4. Safety and efficacy have not been established in clients with a history of seizures or underlying hematologic disease (e.g., hy-

cell anemia).

5. Use with caution in clients with porphyria and preexisting vascular disease.
6. *Do not* give with any other drug solutions.
7. A hemoglobin rise of more than 1 gram/dL over 2 weeks may contribute to increased mortality, serious CV and thromboembolic events.
8. IV usually given as a bolus 3 times per week. May be given into venous line at end of dialysis procedure to obviate need for additional venous access.
9. During hemodialysis, may require increased anticoagulation with heparin to prevent clotting of artificial kidney.
10. Supplemental iron and vitamins are administered to enhance drug effects; take as directed.
11. Must continue to follow prescribed dietary and dialysis recommendations; schedule activities to permit rest periods. Monitor BP and keep record.
12. Do not perform tasks that require mental alertness until drug effects realized (especially during the first 3 months of therapy).

---

## Escitalopram oxalate
(eh-sye-**TAL**-oh-pram)   C

**Rx:** Lexapro.

**CLASSIFICATION(S):** Antidepressant, selective serotonin reuptake inhibitor

**USES:** (1) Major depressive disorder, including maintenance, as defined in the DSM-IV-TR category. (2) Generalized anxiety disorder. *Investigational:* Panic disorder.

**ACTION/KINETICS:** Inhibits CNS neuronal reuptake of serotonin. Minimal effects on norepinephrine and dopamine reuptake. **Peak plasma levels:** About 5 hr. Absorption is not affected by food. **Steady state:** About 1 week following once-daily dosing. Metabo-

lized in the liver by the CYP3A4 and CYP2C19 isoenzymes. $t_{\frac{1}{2}}$, **terminal:** 27–32 hr. About 7% excreted in the urine.
**SIDE EFFECTS:** Nausea, dry mouth, increased sweating, dizziness, diarrhea, flu-like symptoms, fatigue, insomnia, somnolence, rhinitis, ejaculation disorder. *SUICIDE ATTEMPTS.*

## DOSAGE: Oral Solution; Tablets

*Major depressive illness.*
    **Adults, initial:** 10 mg once daily, including the elderly or those with hepatic impairment. Increase dose to 20 mg, if necessary, after a minimum of 1 week. **Maintenance therapy:** 10 or 20 mg/day for up to 36 weeks after an initial 8 weeks of treatment.

*Generalized anxiety disorder.*
    **Adults, initial:** 10 mg once daily. Dose may be increased to 20 mg once daily after a minimum of 1 week. Efficacy after 8 weeks of treatment has not been determined.

## NEED TO KNOW

1. Do not use in clients taking monoamine oxidase inhibitors or citalopram (Celexa).
2. Use with caution in seizure disorders, in clients with diseases or conditions that produce altered metabolism or hemodynamic responses, in impaired hepatic function, severe renal impairment, and in those taking CNS drugs.
3. There is a risk of clinical worsening and suicidal ideation and behavior, especially at the beginning of drug therapy and during dosage adjustments.
4. Give once daily in the morning or evening with or without food.
5. Discontinuing escitalopram may cause symptoms, including dysphoric mood, irritability, agitation, dizziness, sensory disturbances, anxiety, confusion, headache, lethargy, emotional lability, hypomania, or insomnia. A gradual reduction in dose,

rather than abrupt cessation, is recommended whenever possible.

6. Avoid alcohol, OTC agents, or CNS depressants.
7. May see improvement in 1 to 4 weeks; continue as prescribed.

---

## Esomeprazole Magnesium           B
(es-oh-**MEP**-rah-zole)
**Rx:** Nexium.

**CLASSIFICATION(S):** Proton pump inhibitor
**USES: PO only:** (1) Short-term treatment (4–8 weeks) in the healing and symptomatic resolution of diagnostically confirmed erosive esophagitis. An additional 4- to 8-week course may be instituted for those who have not healed. (2) To maintain symptom resolution and healing of erosive esophagitis. (3) Treatment of heartburn and other symptoms associated with GERD in adults. (4) Reduce occurrence of gastric ulcers associated with continuous NSAID therapy in those at risk for developing gastric ulcers (those 60 years and older and/or documented history of gastric ulcers). (5) In combination with amoxicillin and clarithromycin to treat and eradicate *H. pylori* infection and duodenal ulcer disease (active or history in the past years). (6) Long-term treatment of pathological hypersecretory conditions, including Zollinger-Ellison syndrome. **IV only:** Short-term treatment (up to 10 days) of GERD clients with a history of erosive esophagitis as an alternative to PO therapy when therapy with capsules is not possible or appropriate.
**ACTION/KINETICS:** Suppresses the final step in gastric acid production by inhibiting the $H^+/K^+$-ATPase in the gastric parietal cells. This decreases gastric acid secretion. **Peak plasma levels:** 1.5 hr. Absorption is decreased by food. Extensively metabolized in the liver by the cytochrome P450 enzyme system. **t$\frac{1}{2}$, elimination:** 1–1.5 hr. About 80% excreted as inactive metabolites in the urine with 20% excreted in the feces.
**SIDE EFFECTS:** Headache, diarrhea, nausea, stomach pain, consti-

pation, dry mouth. *GI HEMORRHAGE, LARYNGEAL EDEMA, ANGIOEDEMA, ALLERGIC REACTION, ANAPHYLAXIS.*

## DOSAGE: Capsules, Delayed-Release; Suspension, Delayed-Release

*Healing of erosive esophagitis.*
   **Adults:** 20 or 40 mg once daily for 4–8 weeks. For those who do not heal within 4–8 weeks, consider an additional 4–8 weeks of therapy.

*Maintenance of healing of erosive esophagitis.*
   **Adults:** 20 mg once daily, for up to 6 months.

*Symptomatic GERD.*
   **Adults:** 20 mg once daily for 4 weeks. If symptoms do not resolve completely, consider an additional 4 weeks of therapy.

*Eradication of H. pylori to reduce risk of duodenal ulcer recurrence.*
   **Adults:** Use the following triple therapy: Esomeprazole, 40 mg once daily for 10 days; amoxicillin, 1,000 mg twice a day for 10 days; and clarithromycin, 500 mg twice a day for 10 days.

*Reduce risk of NSAID-associated gastric ulcers.*
   **Adults:** 20 or 40 mg once daily for up to 6 months.

*Pathological hypersecretory conditions, including Zollinger-Ellison syndrome.*
   **Adults:** 40 mg twice daily; adjust dose to needs of client.

## DOSAGE: IV

*GERD with history of erosive esophagitis.*
   **Adults:** 20 or 40 mg given once daily by IV injection (no less than 3 min) or by IV infusion over 10–30 min.

## NEED TO KNOW

1. Symptomatic response does not preclude the presence of gastric malignancy.
2. Esomeprazole may interfere with the absorption of drugs where gastric pH is an important factor in bioavailability (e.g., digoxin, iron salts, ketoconazole).

3. For clients unable to swallow capsules, add one tablespoon of applesauce to an empty bowl. Carefully empty the pellets from the capsule onto the applesauce. Mix the pellets with the applesauce and swallow immediately. Do not use hot applesauce and do not chew or crush the pellets. Do not store the pellet/applesauce mixture for future use.

4. For clients with a nasogastric (NG) tube in place, open the capsules and empty the intact granules into a 60 mL syringe. Mix with 50 mL of water. Replace the plunger and shake the syringe vigorously for 15 seconds. Hold the syringe with the tip up and check for granules remaining in the tip. Attach the syringe to the NG tube and deliver the contents through the NG tube into the stomach. Flush the NG tube with additional water.

5. Do not give esomeprazole IV with any other medication through the same IV site and/or tubing. Always flush the IV line with the diluent both prior to and after administration of the drug.

6. Take the delayed-release capsules whole at least 1 hr before meals.

7. May take antacids.

8. Avoid alcohol and OTC products unless approved.

9. Drug is for short-term use only; it inhibits gastric acid secretion. Side effects of prolonged therapy and suppression of acid secretion alter bacterial colonization and lead to hypochlorhydria and hypergastrinemia, which may lead to an increased risk for gastric tumors.

**Estrogens conjugated, oral (conjugated estrogenic substances)** (**ES**-troh-jens)

**X**

**Rx:** Premarin.

**Estrogens conjugated, parenteral**

**Rx:** Premarin Intravenous.

**Estrogens conjugated, synthetic (A & B)**

**Rx:** Cenestin, Enjuvia.

**Estrogens conjugated, vaginal**

**Rx:** Premarin Vaginal Cream.

**CLASSIFICATION(S):** Estrogen, natural and synthetic

**USES: Conjugated Estrogens, PO:** (1) Moderate to severe vasomotor symptoms due to menopause. (2) Moderate to severe symptoms of vulvar and vaginal atrophy associated with menopause. (3) Prophylaxis of postmenopausal osteoporosis. (4) Palliation of breast cancer in selected women and men with metastatic disease. (5) Palliation only of advanced androgen-dependent prostatic carcinoma. **Conjugated Estrogens, Synthetic, A & B, PO:** (1) Moderate to severe vasomotor symptoms associated with menopause. (2) Vulvar and vaginal atrophy (Synthetic Conjugated Estrogens A). **Conjugated Estrogens, Parenteral:** Abnormal bleeding due to imbalance of hormones and in the absence of disease. **Conjugated Estrogens, Vaginal:** Atrophic vaginitis and kraurosis vulvae associated with menopause.

**ACTION/KINETICS:** Estrogens combine with receptors in the cytoplasm of cells, resulting in an increase in protein synthesis. During menopause, estrogens are used as replacement therapy. Metabolized in the liver and excreted mainly in the urine.

**SIDE EFFECTS: After PO Use:** Abdominal/back pain, asthenia, breast pain, headache, infection, dyspepsia, nausea, arthralgia, pharyngitis, URTI.

**DOSAGE: Tablets** ESTROGENS CONJUGATED, ORAL (PREMARIN)

*Moderate to severe vasomotor symptoms due to menopause, moderate to severe symptoms of vulvar and vaginal atrophy associated with menopause.*

**Adults:** Start with the lowest dose: 1.25 mg/day given cyclically. If the client has not menstruated in 2 or more months, begin therapy on any day; if, however, the client is menstruating, begin therapy on day 5 of bleeding.

*Palliation of mammary carcinoma in men or postmenopausal women.*

**Adults:** 10 mg 3 times per day for at least 90 days.

*Palliation of prostatic carcinoma.*

**Adults:** 1.25–2.5 mg 3 times per day. Effectiveness can be measured by phosphatase determinations and symptomatic improvement.

*Prophylaxis of osteoporosis.*

**Adults:** 0.625 mg/day continuously or cyclically (such as 25 days on, 5 days off). Mainstays of therapy include calcium; exercise and nutrition may be important adjuncts.

**DOSAGE: Tablets** ESTROGENS CONJUGATED, SYNTHETIC A (CENESTIN).

*Moderate to severe vasomotor symptoms due to menopause.*

**Adults, initial:** 0.45 mg daily; **then,** adjust dose based on individual client response. Discontinue as soon as possible. Attempt to discontinue or taper dosage at 3- to 6-month intervals.

*Vulvar and vaginal atrophy.*

**Adults:** 0.3 mg/day.

**DOSAGE: Tablets** ESTROGENS CONJUGATED, SYNTHETIC B (ENJUVIA).

*Moderate to severe vasomotor symptoms due to menopause.*

**Adults, initial:** 0.3 mg daily. Adjust dosage based on individual client response. Periodically reassess dosage.

**DOSAGE: Vaginal Cream** Estrogens conjugated, vaginal (Premarin Vaginal Cream)

*Atrophic vaginitis and kraurosis vulvae associated with menopause.*

**Adults:** ½–2 grams daily for 3 weeks on and 1 week off. Repeat as needed. Attempt to taper the dose or discontinue the medication at 3- to 6-month intervals.

---

### NEED TO KNOW

1. Do not use for prevention of CV disease due to increased risk of MI, stroke, invasive breast cancer, and venous thromboembolism.
2. Use of estrogen replacement therapy for prolonged periods of time may increase the risk of fatal ovarian cancer and an increased risk of endometrial cancer.
3. For all uses, except palliation of mammary and prostatic carcinoma, oral conjugated estrogens are best administered cyclically, 3 weeks on and 1 week off.
4. When estrogen is used for a postmenopausal woman with a uterus, also initiate a progestin to reduce the risk of endometrial cancer. Those without a uterus do not require a progestin.
5. For women who have a uterus, undertake adequate diagnostic measures, such as endometrial sampling, when indicated to rule out malignancy in cases of undiagnosed persistent or recurring abnormal vaginal bleeding.
6. May take with food to decrease GI upset.
7. Review potential risks of prolonged therapy, i.e., endometrial cancer, abnormal blood clotting, gallbladder disease, and breast cancer.

## Eszopiclone
(ess-**ZOP**-eye-klone)
**Rx:** Lunesta.

**CLASSIFICATION(S):** Sedative-hypnotic, nonbenzodiazepine
**USES:** Treatment of insomnia.
**ACTION/KINETICS:** May interfere with GABA-receptor complexes at binding domains located close to or allosterically coupled to benzodiazepine receptors. Rapidly absorbed. **Peak plasma levels:** 1 hr. Extensively metabolized by CYP3A4 and CYP2E1 enzymes; one of the metabolites has hypnotic activity. **t½:** About 6 hr. Excreted in the urine (75%); less than 10% is excreted as the parent drug.
**SIDE EFFECTS:** Unpleasant taste, headache, dizziness, diarrhea, dry mouth, dyspepsia, nervousness, somnolence. *UTERINE/VAGINAL HEMORRHAGE.*

**DOSAGE: Tablets**

*Insomnia.*

**Adults, initial:** 2 mg immediately before bedtime for most nonelderly clients. May be initiated at or raised to 3 mg if indicated, as 3 mg is more effective for sleep maintenance. The recommended starting dose for the elderly is 1 mg immediately before bedtime; dose may be increased to 2 mg if indicated. For the elderly who have difficulty staying asleep, give 2 mg immediately before bedtime. Use a starting dose of 1 mg in severe hepatic impairment.

**NEED TO KNOW**

1. Use with caution in those with diseases that could affect metabolism or hemodynamic responses, in those with compromised respiratory function, in those with signs and symptoms of depression.
2. Do not exceed a starting dose of 1 mg in clients coadministered eszopiclone with potent CYP3A4 inhibitors.

3. Do not crush or break tablets and ensure at least 8 hours before required to be up and active.
4. Use caution; do not perform activities that require mental alertness until drug effects are realized. May experience unpleasant taste, dizziness, drowsiness, lightheadedness, and impaired coordination.
5. Avoid alcohol and OTC agents without provider approval.
6. May experience more sleeping problems after stopping drug for the first one or two nights. With prolonged therapy may experience mild withdrawal symptoms.

---

## Etanercept   B
(eh-**TAN**-er-sept)
**Rx:** Enbrel.

**CLASSIFICATION(S):** Immunomodulator
**USES:** (1) Reduce S&S, delays structural damage, and improves physical function in moderate to severe active rheumatoid arthritis in adults who have had an inadequate response to one or more antirheumatic drugs. May be used in combination with methotrexate, in those who do not respond adequately to methotrexate alone. (2) Reduce signs and symptoms of active ankylosing spondylitis. (3) Reduce signs and symptoms, inhibiting the progression of structural damage of active arthritis, and improving physical function in those with psoriatic arthritis. Can be used in combination with methotrexate in those who do not respond adequately to methotrexate alone. (4) Chronic, moderate to severe plaque psoriasis in adults who are candidates for systemic therapy or phototherapy.
**ACTION/KINETICS:** Binds specifically to tumor necrosis factor (TNF) and blocks its interaction with cell surface TNF receptors. TNF is a cytokine that is involved in normal inflammatory and immune responses. Thus, the drug renders TNF biologically inactive. It is possible for etanercept to affect host defenses against infec-

tions and malignancies since TNF mediates inflammation and modulates cellular immune responses. It may also reverse CHF by decreasing inflammation in the heart. t½: About 102 hr. Individual clients may undergo a two- to five-fold increase in serum levels with repeated dosing.

**SIDE EFFECTS:** URTI, non-URTI, injection site reaction, infection, headache, nausea, dizziness, rash, abdominal pain, cough, pharyngitis, asthenia, peripheral edema. *GI HEMORRHAGE, INTESTINAL PERFORATION, STROKE, SEIZURES, CVA, HEART FAILURE, MI, PANCYTOPENIA, INCLUDING APLASTIC ANEMIA, PULMONARY EMBOLISM, SERIOUS INFECTIONS AND SEPSIS, HYPERSENSITIVITY REACTIONS (INCLUDING ANGIOEDEMA).*

## DOSAGE: SC

*Moderate to severe active rheumatoid arthritis; psoriatic arthritis; ankylosing spondylitis.*

> **Adults:** 50 mg per week given as one SC injection using a 50 mg/mL single-use prefilled syringe, or as two 25-mg injections given either on the same day or 3 or 4 days apart. Doses greater than 50 mg per week are not recommended. Methotrexate, glucocorticoids, salicylates, NSAIDs, or analgesics may be used during treatment.

*Plaque psoriasis in adults.*

> **Adults, initial:** 50 mg given twice weekly (3 or 4 days apart) for 3 months; **then,** reduce dose to 50 mg/week. Starting doses of 25 mg or 50 mg per week were also shown to be effective.

## NEED TO KNOW

1. Do not use in any chronic or localized active infection.
2. Use with caution in the elderly and in those with a history of recurring infections or with a condition that predisposes to infections (e.g., advanced or poorly controlled diabetes). Use with caution in those with preexisting or recent-onset CNS-demyelinating disorders.
3. Clients must enroll with the makers of etanercept so that pharmacies can obtain the product.

4. Some clients treated, without interruption, for 3 years may be able to reduce the dose or stop concomitant therapy with methotrexate or corticosteroids.

5. Do not add other medications to solutions containing etanercept and do not reconstitute with other diluents.

6. Give a 50 mg dose as one SC injection using a 50 mg/mL single-use prefilled syringe or as two 25-mg SC injections using the multiple-use vial. Give the two 25-mg injections either on the same day or 3 or 4 days apart.

7. If self-administering etanercept, the first injection will be performed by the client under the supervision of a qualified health care professional.

8. Always rotate sites for self-injection which include the thigh, abdomen, or upper arm. Give new injections at least 1 inch from the old site and never into areas where the skin is tender, bruised, red, or hard.

9. Report any abdominal pain, S&S of infection, dizziness, SOB, chest pain, rash, or other adverse side effects.

10. The manufacturer maintains an active web site www.enbrel.com with patient support services and information. Additionally may call 1-888-4ENBREL (1-888-436-2735) with questions and support.

---

## Ezetimibe
(eh-**ZET**-eh-myb)

**Rx:** Zetia.

**C**

**CLASSIFICATION(S):** Antihyperlipidemic

**USES:** (1) Primary hypercholesterolemia, either as monotherapy or combination therapy with HMG-CoA reductase inhibitors to reduce elevated total cholesterol, LDL-C, and Apo B. (2) With atorvastatin or simvastatin for homozygous familial hypercholesterolemia as an adjunct to other lipid-lowering treatments. (3) As adjunctive therapy to diet for homozygous sitosterolemia. (4) With fenofibrate as adjunctive therapy to diet to reduce total cholesterol, LDL-C, Apo B, and non–high-density lipoprotein cholesterol in clients with mixed hyperlipidemia.

**ACTION/KINETICS:** Acts by inhibiting the absorption of cholesterol from the small intestine, leading to a decrease in the delivery of cholesterol to the liver. Reduces total cholesterol, LDL cholesterol, Apo B, and triglycerides as well as increases HDL cholesterol. **Peak plasma ezetimibe levels:** 4–12 hr. **t½, parent drug and active metabolite:** 22 hr. After PO administration, is rapidly conjugated to the active phenolic glucuronide in the small intestine and liver. Mainly excreted through the feces with smaller amounts through the urine.

**SIDE EFFECTS:** Back/abdominal pain, diarrhea, arthralgia, sinusitis, coughing, pharyngitis. *PANCREATITIS.*

---

**DOSAGE: Tablets**

*Primary hypercholesterolemia, homozygous familial hypercholesterolemia, homozygous sitosterolemia, with fenofibrate in mixed hyperlipidemia.*

**Adults:** 10 mg once daily with or without food.

---

**NEED TO KNOW**

1. Do not use in active liver disease or unexplained persistent elevations in serum transaminases.
2. Place client on a standard cholesterol-lowering diet before therapy and for duration of treatment.
3. Give at least 2 hr before or at least 4 hr after giving a bile sequestrant.
4. Before initiating therapy exclude or, if appropriate, treat secondary causes for dyslipidemia (e.g., diabetes, hypothyroidism, obstructive liver disease, chronic renal failure, drugs that increase LDL-C and decrease HDL-C).
5. Take daily as directed with or without food. Avoid taking with antacids; reduces drug effect.
6. Report any S&S of infections, unexplained muscle pain, tenderness/weakness (especially if accompanied by fever or mal-

aise), surgery, trauma, or metabolic disorders. Report as scheduled for lab tests, eye exam, and follow up.

7. Review importance of following a low-cholesterol diet, regular exercise, low alcohol consumption, and not smoking in the overall plan to reduce serum cholesterol levels and inhibit progression of CAD.

## Ezetimibe and Simvastatin
(eh-**ZET**-eh-myb, **sim**-vah-**STAH**-tin)
**Rx:** Vytorin 10/10, 10/20, 10/40, or 10/80.

**CLASSIFICATION(S):** Combination antihyperlipidemic
**USES:** (1) Adjunctive therapy to diet to reduce elevated total-C, LDL-C, Apo B, triglycerides, and non-HDL-C and to increase HDL-C in clients with primary (heterozygous familial or non-familial) hypercholesterolemia or mixed hyperlipidemia. (2) Reduction of elevated total-C and LDL-C in clients with homozygous familial hypercholesterolemia, as an adjunct to other lipid-lowering treatments (or if such treatments are not available).
**ACTION/KINETICS:** Ezetimibe reduces blood cholesterol by inhibiting absorption of cholesterol by the small intestine, leading to a decrease of hepatic cholesterol stores and an increased clearance of cholesterol from the blood. Simvastatin decreases cholesterol by inhibiting conversion of HMG-CoA to mevalonate, an early step in the biosynthesis of cholesterol. Also, simvastatin reduces VLDL and triglycerides and increases HDL-C. Ezetimibe is absorbed and converted to the active exetimibe-glucuronide. High fat or non-fat meals have no effect on the extent of absorption. Ezetimibe is metabolized in the small intestine and liver by glucuroide conjugation and excreted in both the feces and urine. Simvastatin undergoes extensive first-pass liver metabolism and is mainly excreted in the bile.
**SIDE EFFECTS:** Headache, myalgia, URTI, influenza, abdominal pain, diarrhea, arthralgia, back pain, sinusitis, chest pain.

### DOSAGE: Tablets

*Primary hypercholesterolemia.*

**Adults, usual, initial:** 10/20 mg/day. Beginning with 10/10 mg/day may be considered for those requiring less aggressive LDL-C reductions. Those requiring a larger LDL-C reduction (greater than 55%) may be started on 10/40 mg/day. After initiation or titration of Vytorin, lipid levels may be analyzed after 2 or more weeks; adjust dosage, if necessary. **Dose range:** 10/10 mg/day through 10/80 mg/day.

*Homozygous familial hypercholesterolemia.*

**Adults:** 10/40 mg/day or 10/80 mg/day, with other lipid-lowering treatments (e.g., LDL apheresis).

---

### NEED TO KNOW

1. All strengths contain ezetimibe, 10 mg with either 10 mg, 20 mg, 40 mg, or 80 mg simvastatin.
2. Use not recommended with moderate or severe hepatic insufficiency.
3. Prior to beginning therapy with Vytorin, secondary causes for dyslipidemia (i.e., diabetes, hypothyroidism, obstructive liver disease, chronic renal failure, and drugs that increase LDL-C and decrease HDL-C) should be excluded or, if appropriate, treated.
4. Place client on a standard cholesterol-lowering diet before giving Vytorn; continue the diet during Vytorin treatment.
5. In severe renal insufficiency, do not begin Vytorin unless client has tolerated treatment with simvastatin, at a dose of 5 mg or higher.
6. If given with bile acid sequestrants, give Vytorin either 2 hr or more before or 4 hr or more after giving the bile acid sequestrant.
7. Take as a single dose in the evening, with or without food.
8. May cause visual changes or drowsiness.
9. Avoid grapefruit and grapefruit juice; may increase drug concentrations and adverse effects.

10. Report any new onset muscle pain, weakness, tenderness, or fever.
11. Avoid alcohol: may increase risk of liver problems.

## Finasteride
(fin-**AS**-teh-ride)
**Rx:** Propecia, Proscar.

**X**

**CLASSIFICATION(S):** Androgen hormone inhibitor
**USES:** (1) Improve symptoms of benign prostatic hyperplasia (BPH) to reduce risk of acute urinary infection and reduce risk for surgery and prostatectomy (Proscar only). (2) In combination with doxazosin to decrease risk of benign prostatic hypertrophy symptoms from progressing over time.
**ACTION/KINETICS:** Is a specific inhibitor of 5-α-reductase, the enzyme that converts testosterone to the active 5-α-dihydrotestosterone (DHT). Thus, there are significant decreases in serum and tissue DHT levels, resulting in rapid regression of prostate tissue and an increase in urine flow and symptomatic improvement. Also a decrease in scalp DHT levels. Well absorbed after PO administration. **Elimination t½:** 6 hr in clients 45–60 years of age and 8 hr in clients over 70 years of age. Slow accumulation after multiple dosing. Metabolized in the liver and excreted through both the urine and feces.
**SIDE EFFECTS:** Impotence, decreased libido, postural hypotension, dizziness, asthenia, headache, ejaculation disorder.

## DOSAGE: Tablets

*Benign prostatic hyperplasia.*
**Adults:** 5 mg/day, with or without meals.

## NEED TO KNOW

1. Use with caution in clients with impaired liver function.
2. At least 6–12 months of therapy may be required to deter-

mine whether a beneficial response has been achieved for BPH.

3. Do not adjust dosage in the elderly or in those with impaired renal function.
4. The following symptoms of BPH should show improvement with continued drug therapy: hesitancy, feelings of incomplete bladder emptying, interruption of urinary stream, impairment of size and force of urinary stream, and terminal urinary dribbling.
5. May lower PSA levels (prostate-specific antigen: a blood screening study to detect prostate cancer) even in the presence of prostate cancer.
6. Decreased volume of ejaculate may occur but does not interfere with sexual function. Impotence and decreased libido may occur.
7. Interruption of therapy will reverse effects within 12 months and BPH symptoms will return.

## Fluoxetine hydrochloride B
(flew-**OX**-eh-teen)
**Rx:** Prozac, Prozac Pulvules, Prozac Weekly.

CLASSIFICATION(S): Antidepressant, selective serotonin reuptake inhibitor
USES: **Prozac:** (1) Major depressive disorder as defined in the DSM-IV. (2) Obsessive-compulsive disorder (OCD) as defined in the DSM-III-R. (3) Panic disorder with or without agoraphobia as defined in DSM-IV.
ACTION/KINETICS: Antidepressant effect likely due to inhibition of CNS neuronal uptake of serotonin and to a lesser extent norepinephrine and dopamine. Results in increased levels of serotonin in synapses. Metabolized in the liver to norfluoxetine, a metabolite with equal potency to fluoxetine. Norfluoxetine is further metabolized by the liver to inactive metabolites that are excreted by the kidneys. **Time to peak plasma levels:** 6–8 hr. **Peak plasma con-**

**centrations:** 15–55 ng/mL. **t½, fluoxetine:** 1–6 days; **t½, norfluoxetine:** 4–16 days. **Time to steady state:** About 4 weeks. Active drug maintained in the body for weeks after withdrawal.

**SIDE EFFECTS:** Insomnia, nausea, somnolence, nervousness, anxiety, tremor, diarrhea/loose stools, anorexia, dry mouth. *SOME CLIENTS MAY EXPERIENCE SEIZURES OR ATTEMPT SUICIDE.*

**DOSAGE: Capsules; Capsules, Delayed Release; Oral Solution; Tablets** PROZAC (ALL FORMS)

*Major depressive disorder.*

**Adults, initial:** 20 mg/day in the morning. If clinical improvement is not observed after several weeks, the dose may be increased to a maximum of 80 mg/day in two equally divided doses. For weekly dosing for stabilized clients requiring maintenance therapy, can use Prozac Weekly (90 mg delayed-release capsule), given 7 days after the last 20 mg dose. If satisfactory response is not maintained, reestablish a daily dosing regimen.

*OCD.*

**Adults, initial:** 20 mg/day in the morning. If improvement is not significant after several weeks, the dose may be increased. Full effect may be delayed until 5 weeks of treatment or longer. **Usual dosage range:** 20–60 mg/day; the total daily dosage should not exceed 80 mg. Adjust dose to maintain client on lowest effective dosage. **Maintenance:** Clients have been continued on therapy for an additional 6 months after an initial 13 weeks of treatment, without loss of efficacy. Adjust dose to maintain on lowest effective dose; periodically reassess to determine need for continued treatment.

*Panic disorder.*

**Adults, initial:** 10 mg/day. After 1 week, increase the dose to 20 mg/day. A dose increase may be considered after several weeks if no improvement is noted. Doses above 60 mg/day have not been evaluated in panic disorders.

1. Do not use thioridazine with fluoxetine or within a minimum of 5 weeks after fluoxetine has been discontinued.
2. A lower dose or less frequent dosing should be considered for those with impaired hepatic function, elderly clients, those with concurrent diseases, or those who are taking multiple medications.
3. Divide doses greater than 20 mg/day and give in the a.m. and at noon.
4. If doses lower than 20 mg are necessary, the drug may be emptied from the capsule into cranberry, orange, or apple juice; this should not be refrigerated (is stable for 2 weeks).
5. The maximum therapeutic effect may not be observed until 4–5 weeks after beginning therapy.
6. Elderly clients, clients taking multiple medications, and those with liver or kidney dysfunction should take lower or less frequent doses.
7. Allow 14 days to elapse between discontinuing a MAOI and starting fluoxetine therapy; also, allow 5 weeks or more to elapse between stopping fluoxetine and starting a MAOI.
8. May be taken with food to decrease chance of stomach upset.
9. Report side effects, especially rashes, hives, increased anxiety, loss of appetite, or lack of response. Use reliable birth control during therapy.
10. Usually takes 1 month to note any significant benefits from therapy.

---

**Fluvastatin sodium**      **X**
(flu-vah-**STAH**-tin)
**Rx:** Lescol, Lescol XL.

**CLASSIFICATION(S):** Antihyperlipidemic, HMG-CoA reductase inhibitor
**USES:** (1) Reduce elevated total and LDL cholesterol, Apo-B, and triglyceride levels and to increase HDL cholesterol in clients with

primary hypercholesterolemia (heterozygous familial and nonfamilial) and mixed dyslipidemia (Fredrickson type IIa and IIb) whose response to diet and other nondrug measures has been inadequate. The lipid-lowering effects of fluvastatin are enhanced when it is combined with a bile-acid binding resin or with niacin. (2) To slow the progression of coronary atherosclerosis in coronary heart disease as part of a treatment plan to lower total and LDL cholesterol to target levels. (3) Reduce the risk of undergoing coronary revascularization procedures in those with coronary heart disease. **ACTION/KINETICS:** Decreases cholesterol, triglycerides, VLDL, and HDL and increases HDL. Undergoes extensive first-pass metabolism by CYP2C9. Metabolized in the liver with 90% excreted through the feces and 5% through the urine. **t½:** Less than 3 hr for immediate-release and about 9 hr for extended-release. **SIDE EFFECTS:** UTRI, dysgeusia, diarrhea, abdominal pain/cramps, N&V, constipation, myalgia, back pain, arthralgia, rhinitis, pharyngitis, influenza, accidental trauma.

**DOSAGE:** Capsules; Tablets, Extended-Release

*Hypercholesterolemia and mixed dyslipidemia. Antihyperlipidemic to slow progression of coronary atherosclerosis. Secondary prevention of coronary events.*

**Adults: For those requiring LDL cholesterol reduction to 25% or more, initial,** 40 mg as one capsule in the evening or 80 mg as one tablet any time of day. Or, 80 mg in divided doses using the 40 mg capsule twice a day. **For those requiring LDL cholesterol reduction to less than 25%, initial:** 20 mg. **Dose range:** 20–80 mg/day.

*Slow progression of coronary atherosclerosis in coronary heart disease.*

**Adults:** 40 mg twice a day, initiated shortly after a first percutaneous coronary intervention procedure.

1. Use with caution in clients with severe renal impairment, a history of liver disease, or heavy alcohol consumption.
2. Place on standard cholesterol-lowering diet before receiving fluvastatin; continue diet during therapy.
3. Maximum reductions of LDL cholesterol are usually seen within 4 weeks.
4. To avoid fluvastatin binding to a bile-acid binding resin (if given together), give the fluvastatin at bedtime and the resin at least 2 hr before.
5. May be taken with or without food; usually consumed with the evening meal.
6. Report muscle pain or weakness, especially with fever or severe fatigue, or other adverse effects. Keep scheduled lab visits.
7. Avoid alcohol consumption.

## Fluvoxamine maleate (flu-**VOX**-ah-meen) ■ C

**CLASSIFICATION(S):** Antidepressant, selective serotonin reuptake inhibitor

**USES:** Obsessive-compulsive disorder (OCD) as defined in DSM-III-R for adults.

**ACTION/KINETICS:** Minimal to no anticholinergic or sedative effects; no orthostatic hypotension. **Maximum plasma levels:** 3–8 hr. **t½:** 13.6–15.6 hr. **Peak plasma concentration:** 88–546 ng/mL. **Time to reach steady state:** About 7 days. Elderly clients manifest higher mean plasma levels and a decreased clearance. Metabolized in the liver and about 94% excreted through the urine.

**SIDE EFFECTS:** Nausea, insomnia, somnolence, headache, nervousness, asthenia, dizziness, diarrhea/loose stools, dyspepsia, dry mouth, constipation, URTI. CONVULSION, GI HEMORRHAGE, CARDIOMYOPATHY, HEART FAILURE, MI, SUICIDE ATTEMPT.

## DOSAGE: Tablets

*Obsessive-compulsive disorder.*

**Adults, initial:** 50 mg at bedtime; **then,** increase the dose in 50 mg increments q 4–7 days, as tolerated, until a maximum benefit is reached, not to exceed 300 mg/day. Give total daily doses greater than 100 mg in 2 divided doses; if doses are unequal, give the larger dose at bedtime. **Maintenance:** Although efficacy has not been documented beyond 10 weeks, consider continuation in a responding client since OCD is a chronic condition. Adjust dose to maintain the lowest effective dosage; periodically reassess to determine need for continued treatment.

### NEED TO KNOW

1. Do not use with alosetron, pimozide, thioridazine, or tizanidine.
2. Initial and incremental doses may need to be lower in geriatric clients and with impaired hepatic function.
3. May initially experience N&V; should subside.
4. May cause dizziness and drowsiness. Do not perform activities that require mental or physical alertness until drug effects realized.
5. Report any rash, hives, or unusual itching or bleeding; increased depression or suicide ideations.
6. Avoid alcohol and other drugs or herbals without approval. Smoking may reduce drug effectiveness.

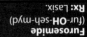

# Furosemide
(fur-OH-seh-myd) **C**

**Rx:** Lasix.

**CLASSIFICATION(S):** Diuretic, loop

**USES:** (1) Edema associated with CHF, nephrotic syndrome, hepat-

to treat hypertension in conjunction with spironolactone, triamterene, and other diuretics *except* ethacrynic acid.

**ACTION/KINETICS:** Inhibits the reabsorption of sodium and chloride in the proximal and distal tubules as well as the ascending loop of Henle; this results in the excretion of sodium, chloride, and, to a lesser degree, potassium and bicarbonate ions. Diuretic action is independent of changes in clients' acid-base balance. **Onset:** PO, IM: 30–60 min; **IV:** 5 min. **Peak:** PO, IM: 1–2 hr; **IV:** 20–60 min. **t½:** About 2 hr after PO use. **Duration:** PO, IM: 6–8 hr; **IV:** 2 hr. Metabolized in the liver and excreted through the urine. May be effective for clients resistant to thiazides and for those with reduced GFRs.

**SIDE EFFECTS:** Jaundice, tinnitus, hearing impairment, hypotension, water/electrolyte depletion, pancreatitis, abdominal pain, dizziness, anemia. *AGRANULOCYTOSIS, RARELY, APLASTIC ANEMIA.*

**DOSAGE: Oral Solution; Tablets**

*Edema.*

**Adults, initial:** 20–80 mg/day as a single dose. For resistant cases, dosage can be increased by 20–40 mg q 6–8 hr until desired diuretic response is attained. Maximum daily dose should not exceed 600 mg.

*Hypertension.*

**Adults, initial:** 40 mg twice a day. Adjust dosage depending on response.

*CHF and chronic renal failure.*

**Adults:** 2–2.5 grams/day.

*Antihypercalcemic.*

**Adults:** 120 mg/day in one to three doses.

**DOSAGE: IM; IV**

*Edema.*

**Adults, initial:** 20–40 mg; if response inadequate after 2 hr, increase dose in 20-mg increments.

*Antihypercalcemic.*
**Adults:** 80–100 mg for severe cases; dose may be repeated q 1–2 hr if needed.

## DOSAGE: IV

*Acute pulmonary edema.*
**Adults:** 40 mg slowly over 1–2 min; if response inadequate after 1 hr, give 80 mg slowly over 1–2 min. Concomitant oxygen and digitalis may be used.

*CHF, chronic renal failure.*
**Adults:** 2–2.5 grams/day. For IV bolus injections, the maximum should not exceed 1 gram/day given over 30 min.

*Hypertensive crisis, normal renal function.*
**Adults:** 40–80 mg.

*Hypertensive crisis with pulmonary edema or acute renal failure.*
**Adults:** 100–200 mg.

## NEED TO KNOW

1. Furosemide is a potent diuretic. Excess amounts can lead to profound diuresis with water and electrolyte depletion.
2. Never use with ethacrynic acid.
3. Geriatric clients may be more sensitive to the usual adult dose. Allergic reactions may be seen in clients who show hypersensitivity to sulfonamides.
4. Give 2–4 days per week.
5. Food decreases bioavailability of furosemide and ultimately the degree of diuresis.
6. If used with other antihypertensives, reduce dose of other agents by at least 50% when furosemide is added in order to prevent an excessive drop in BP.
7. Give IV injections slowly over 1–2 min.
8. A precipitate may form if mixed with gentamicin, netilmicin, or milrinone in either D5W or NSS.
9. Take in the morning on an empty stomach to enhance absorption and avoid interruption of sleep. May take with food

activities.
10. Immediately report any muscle weakness/cramps, dizziness, ringing in the ears, sore throat, fever, severe abdominal pain, numbness, or tingling.
11. Drug may cause BP drop. Change positions from lying to standing slowly.
12. Consult provider before taking excessive aspirin for any reason. Salicylate intoxication occurs at lower levels than normal because of competition at the renal excretory sites.
13. Supplement diet with vegetables and fruits that are high in potassium (bananas, oranges, peaches, dried dates) if oral supplements are not prescribed. Those on a salt-restricted diet should not increase salt intake; NSAIDs and alpha blockers may also cause sodium retention.

## Glimepiride
(GLYE-meh-pye-ride)

**C**

**Rx: Amaryl.**

**CLASSIFICATION(S):** Antidiabetic, oral; second generation sulfonylurea

**USES:** (1) As an adjunct to diet and exercise to lower blood glucose in non-insulin-dependent diabetes mellitus (type 2 diabetes mellitus) whose hyperglycemia can not be controlled by diet and exercise alone. (2) In combination with insulin to decrease blood glucose in those whose hyperglycemia cannot be controlled by diet and exercise in combination with an oral hypoglycemic drug. (3) In combination with metformin (Glucophage) if control is not reached with diet, exercise, and either hypoglycemic alone.

**ACTION/KINETICS:** Lowers blood glucose by stimulating the release of insulin from functioning pancreatic beta cells and by increasing the sensitivity of peripheral tissues to insulin. Completely absorbed from the GI tract within 1 hr. **Onset:** 2–3 hr. **t½, serum:**

About 9 hr. **Duration:** 24 hr. Completely metabolized in the liver and metabolites are excreted through both the urine and feces. **SIDE EFFECTS:** Hypoglycemia, dizziness, weakness, headache, blurred vision. *APLASTIC ANEMIA.*

## DOSAGE: Tablets

*Type 2 diabetes.*

**Adults, initial:** 1–2 mg once daily, given with breakfast or the first main meal. The initial dose should be 1 mg in those sensitive to hypoglycemic drugs, in those with impaired renal or hepatic function, and in elderly, debilitated, or malnourished clients. The maximum initial dose is 2 mg or less daily. **Maintenance:** 1–4 mg once daily up to a maximum of 8 mg once daily. After a dose of 2 mg is reached, increase the dose in increments of 2 mg or less at 1- to 2-week intervals (determined by the blood glucose response). **When combined with insulin therapy:** 8 mg once daily with the first main meal with low-dose insulin. The fasting glucose level for beginning combination therapy is greater than 150 mg/dL glucose in the plasma or serum. After starting with low-dose insulin, upward adjustments of insulin can be done about weekly as determined by frequent fasting blood glucose determinations.

*Type 2 diabetes—transfer from other hypoglycemic agents.*

**Adults:** When transferring clients to glimepiride, no transition period is required. However, observe clients closely for 1 to 2 weeks for hypoglycemia when being transferred from longer half-life sulfonylureas (e.g., chlorpropamide) to glimepiride.

## NEED TO KNOW

1. Do not use in diabetic ketoacidosis with or without coma.
2. The use of oral hypoglycemic drugs has been associated with increased CV mortality compared with treatment with diet alone or diet plus insulin.
3. Continue regular exercise and dietary restrictions, BP and cholesterol control in addition to drug therapy.

4. Avoid alcohol and direct of artificial sun exposure. Report any adverse effects.

---

## Glipizide        C
(**GLIP**-ih-zyd)
**Rx:** Glipizide Extended-Release, Glucotrol, Glucotrol XL.

**CLASSIFICATION(S):** Antidiabetic, oral; second generation sulfonylurea

**USES:** Adjunct to diet for control of hyperglycemia in clients with non-insulin-dependent diabetes mellitus (type 2 diabetes). Begin therapy when diet alone has been unsuccessful in controlling hyperglycemia.

**ACTION/KINETICS:** Lowers blood glucose by stimulating the release of insulin from functioning pancreatic beta cells and by increasing the sensitivity of peripheral tissues to insulin. Also has mild diuretic effects. **Onset:** 1–3 hr. **t½:** 2–4 hr. **Duration:** 10–24 hr. Metabolized in liver to inactive metabolites, which are excreted through the kidneys.

**SIDE EFFECTS:** Hypoglycemia, headache, dizziness, hives, skin rash, jaundice.

---

**DOSAGE: Tablets, Immediate-Release**

*Type 2 diabetes.*

**Adults, initial:** 5 mg 30 min before breakfast; **then,** adjust dosage by 2.5–5 mg every few days, depending on the blood glucose response, until adequate control is achieved. **Maintenance:** 15–40 mg/day; divide total daily doses over 15 mg/day. Older clients or those with liver disease should begin with 2.5 mg.

**DOSAGE: Tablets, Extended-Release**

*Type 2 diabetes.*

**Adults (including geriatric clients), initial:** 5 mg with breakfast. Monitor response to therapy by measuring HbA1c at 3-month intervals. Dose can be increased to 10 mg if response is inadequate. **Maintenance:** 5 or 10 mg once daily; some may require 20 mg/day (maximum).

## NEED TO KNOW

1. Divide maintenance doses greater than 15 mg/day; give before the morning and evening meals. Total daily doses of 30 mg or more may be given safely on twice daily dosing.

2. No transition period needed when transferring to extended-release tablets from other oral antidiabetic drugs. Observe for 1–2 weeks if transferred from long half-life sulfonylureas (e.g., chlorpropamide) to extended-release glipizide due to overlapping effects.

3. When transferring from insulin dose of less than 20 units/day, insulin may be discontinued abruptly. When transferring from an insulin dose of greater than 20 units/day, reduce insulin dose by 50%; further reduce depending on response. The initial glipizide dose when transferring from insulin is 5 mg/day.

4. Take 30 min before or with meals (to lessen chance of stomach upset). Do not chew or crush extended release form (i.e., Glucotrol XL).

5. Report CNS side effects: drowsiness, headache; check fingerstick.

6. May have anorexia, constipation, diarrhea, vomiting, stomach pain. Report if severe, record weight, I&O.

7. Report if skin reactions occur. Avoid exposure to direct/artificial light; use sunscreen, sunglasses, protective clothing when outdoors.

8. Avoid alcohol or OTC agents without approval.

# Glyburide
## (GLYE-byou-ryd)
**Rx:** Diaβeta, Glynase PresTab, Micronase.

**B**

**CLASSIFICATION(S):** Antidiabetic, oral; second generation sulfonylurea

**USES:** Non-insulin-dependent diabetes mellitus (type 2 diabetes) whose hyperglycemia cannot be controlled by diet alone. May be used with metformin when diet and glyburide or diet and metformin alone do not provide adequate control.

**ACTION/KINETICS:** Lowers blood glucose by stimulating the release of insulin from functioning pancreatic beta cells and by increasing the sensitivity of peripheral tissues to insulin. Has a mild diuretic effect. **Onset, nonmicronized:** 2–4 hr; **micronized:** 1 hr. **t½, nonmicronized:** 10 hr; **micronized:** Approximately 4 hr. **Time to peak levels:** 4 hr. **Duration, nonmicronized:** 16–24 hr; **micronized:** 12–24 hr. Metabolized in liver to weakly active metabolites. Excreted in bile (50%) and through the kidneys (50%). Micronized glyburide (3 mg tablets) produces serum levels that are not bioequivalent to those from nonmicronized glyburide (5 mg tablets).

**SIDE EFFECTS:** Hypoglycemia, nausea, epigastric distress, heartburn, allergic skin reactions, blurred vision.

**DOSAGE: Tablets, Nonmicronized** DIAβETA/MICRONASE

*Type 2 diabetes.*

**Adults, initial:** 2.5–5 mg/day given with breakfast (or the first main meal); **then,** increase by 2.5 mg at weekly intervals to achieve the desired response. **Maintenance:** 1.25–20 (maximum) mg/day. Clients sensitive to sulfonylureas should start with 1.25 mg/day.

**DOSAGE: Tablets, Micronized** GLYNASE PRESTAB

*Type 2 diabetes.*

**Adults, initial:** 1.5–3 mg/day given with breakfast (or the first main meal). Those sensitive to sulfonylureas should start with

0.75 mg/day. Increase by no more than 1.5 mg at weekly intervals to achieve the desired response. **Maintenance:** 0.75–12 (maximum) mg/day.

**NEED TO KNOW**

1. For best results, administer 30 min prior to meals.
2. To avoid hypoglycemic reactions, the initial and maintenance doses should be conservative in the elderly, the debilitated, or in those with impaired hepatic or renal function.
3. If daily dosage of the nonmicronized product exceeds 15 mg or the micronized product exceeds 6 mg, dividing the dose and giving before the morning and evening meals may be more effective.
4. When transferring from oral hypoglycemics, other than chlorpropamide, no transition and no initial priming dose are required. When transferring from chlorpropamide, use caution for the first 2 weeks due to the long duration of action of chlorpropamide and possible overlapping drug effects.
5. Add glyburide tablets gradually to the dosing regimen of those who have not responded to the maximum dose of metformin monotherapy after 4 weeks.
6. Use the following guidelines when transferring from insulin to glyburide:
   - Insulin dose less than 20 units/day, start with 1.5–3 mg/day micronized or 2.5–5 mg/day nonmicronized glyburide. Insulin may be discontinued abruptly.
   - Insulin dose from 20–40 units/day, start with 3 mg/day micronized or 5 mg/day nonmicronized glyburide. Insulin may be discontinued abruptly.
   - Insulin dose more than 40 units/day, start with 3 mg/day micronized or 5 mg/day nonmicronized glyburide. Reduce insulin dose by 50%; reduce further as determined by response. Consider hospitalization during the transition.
7. Avoid alcohol or OTC agents without approval.

**CLASSIFICATION(S):** Antidiabetic, oral

**USES:** (1) As an adjunct to diet and exercise, and as initial therapy, to improve glycemic control in non-insulin-dependent diabetes mellitus (type 2 diabetes) in those who can not be controlled satisfactorily with diet and exercise alone. (2) Second-line therapy when diet, exercise, and initial therapy with a sulfonylurea or metformin do not provide adequate control in those with type 2 diabetes. If additional control is needed, a thiazolidinedione may be added to Glucovance therapy.

**ACTION/KINETICS:** Glyburide stimulates release of insulin from the pancreas, which is dependent upon functioning pancreatic beta islets. Extrapancreatic effects may also be involved in the long-term effectiveness of glyburide. Metformin decreases hepatic glucose production, decreases intestinal absorption of glucose, and improves insulin sensitivity by increasing peripheral glucose uptake and utilization. Thus the mechanisms are complementary. Glyburide is rapidly absorbed; **peak levels:** 4 hr. Food decreases the extent and slightly delays the absorption of metformin. Glyburide is significantly bound to plasma proteins while metformin is negligibly bound. Steady state metformin levels are reached within 24–48 hr. **Glyburide, $t^{1}\!/_{2}$, terminal:** About 10 hr; excreted as metabolites in the bile and urine (about 50% by each route). Metformin is excreted unchanged in the urine; **$t^{1}\!/_{2}$, elimination:** About 17.6 hr.

**SIDE EFFECTS:** URTI, diarrhea, hypoglycemia, headache, N&V, abdominal pain, dizziness.

---

**DOSAGE: Tablets**

*Type 2 diabetes, initial therapy.*

   **Adults, initial:** 1.25 mg/250 mg once a day with a meal. In those with baseline HbA1c more than 9% or an FBG more than 200 mg/dL, give an initial dose of 1.25 mg/250 mg twice a day with the morning and evening meals. Do not use Glucovance, 5 mg/500 mg, as initial therapy due to the increased risk of hypoglycemia. Make dosage increases in increments of 1.25 mg/250 mg per day every 2 weeks up to the minimum effective dose needed to control blood glucose, not to exceed 20 mg glyburide/2,000 mg metformin daily.

*Type 2 diabetes, in previously treated clients (second-line therapy).*
**Adults, initial:** Either 2.5 mg/500 mg or 5 mg/500 mg twice a day with the morning and evening meals. Titrate the daily dose in increments of no more than 5 mg/500 mg, up to the minimum effective dose to achieve adequate blood glucose control or a maximum dose of 20 mg/2,000 mg daily.

## NEED TO KNOW

1. Lactic acidosis is a rare, but serious, metabolic complication that can occur due to metformin accumulation during treatment with Glucovance.
2. Because impaired hepatic function may significantly limit the ability to clear lactate, Glucovance should generally be avoided in clients with clinical or laboratory evidence of hepatic disease.
3. Clients should be cautioned against excessive alcohol intake, either acute or chronic, when taking Glucovance, since alcohol potentiates the effects of metformin on lactate metabolism.
4. Do not use in renal disease or renal dysfunction (including that due to shock, acute MI, septicemia), CHF requiring pharmacologic treatment, acute or chronic metabolic acidosis (including diabetic ketoacidosis, with or without coma), and known hypersensitivity to glyburide or metformin.
5. To avoid the risk of hypoglycemia, generally do not titrate to the maximum dose of Glucovance in the elderly, debilitated, or malnourished client.
6. For clients not adequately controlled on Glucovance, a thiazolidinedione can be added to therapy. When a thiazolidinedione is added, the current dose of Glucovance can be contin-

ued and the thiazolidinedione added at its recommended starting dose.

7. Temporarily discontinue Glucovance in those undergoing radiologic studies involving intravascular administration of iodinated contrast materials; use of such products may result in acute alteration of renal function.

8. Take with meals as directed. Do not take if meal skipped.

9. May cause drowsiness, dizziness, blurred vision; avoid activities that require mental alertness until drug effects realized.

10. Report symptoms of lactic acidosis: weakness, increasing sleepiness, slow heart rate, cold feeling, muscle pain, shortness of breath, stomach pain, feeling light-headed, fainting.

11. May cause photosensitivity; avoid prolonged sun exposure and use protection if exposed.

## Hydrochlorothiazide B
(hy-droh-klor-oh-**THIGH**-ah-zyd)

**Rx:** Ezide, Hydro-Par, HydroDIURIL, Microzide Capsules.

**CLASSIFICATION(S):** Diuretic, thiazide

**USES:** (1) Hypertension. Hydrochlorothiazide is a component of a large number of combination drugs used to treat hypertension. (2) Diuretic to treat edema due to CHF, nephrosis, nephritis, renal failure, PMS, hepatic cirrhosis, corticosteroid or estrogen therapy. (3) Microzide is available for once-daily, low-dose treatment for hypertension.

**ACTION/KINETICS:** Promote the excretion of sodium and chloride, and thus water, by the distal renal tubule. Also increases excretion of potassium and to a lesser extent, bicarbonate. The antihypertensive activity is thought to be due to direct dilation of the arterioles, as well as to a reduction in the total fluid volume of the body and altered sodium balance. **Onset:** 2 hr. **Peak effect:** 4–6 hr. **Duration:** 6–12 hr. **t½:** 5.6–14.8 hr. Hydrochlorothiazide is not metabolized but is eliminated rapidly by the kidney.

**SIDE EFFECTS:** Orthostatic hypotension, hypokalemia, weakness,

headache, diarrhea, dizziness, gastric upset/irritation/cramping.
*TOXIC EPIDERMAL NECROLYSIS, STEVENS-JOHNSON SYNDROME, ANAPHYLACTIC REAC-TIONS, RESPIRATORY DISTRESS INCLUDING PNEUMONITIS AND PULMONARY EDEMA.*

## DOSAGE: Capsules; Oral Solution; Tablets
*Diuretic.*
   **Adults, initial:** 25–200 mg/day for several days until dry weight is reached; **then,** 25–100 mg/day or intermittently. Some clients may require up to 200 mg/day.

*Antihypertensive.*
   **Adults, initial:** 25 mg/day as a single dose. The dose may be increased to 50 mg/day in one to two daily doses. Doses greater than 50 mg may cause significant reductions in serum potassium.

NEED TO KNOW
   1. Geriatric clients may be more sensitive to the usual adult dose.
   2. Divide daily doses in excess of 100 mg.
   3. When used with other antihypertensives, hydrochlorothiazide dose is usually not more than 50 mg.
   4. Take in the a.m. with a glass of orange juice to prevent night-time urinary frequency. May take with food if GI upset. Report side effects or lack of response.
   5. Avoid alcohol, OTC agents, and prolonged sun exposure; may cause delayed (10–14 day) photosensitivity reaction.
   6. With diabetes, monitor BS and potassium closely; may cause glucose intolerance.

**CLASSIFICATION(S):** Bone growth regulator, bisphosphonate

**USES: Tablets:** Prophylaxis of postmenopausal osteoporosis in women who are at risk of developing osteoporosis and for whom the desired clinical outcome is to maintain bone mass and reduce the risk of fracture. **Injection/Tablets:** Treatment of postmenopausal osteoporosis to increase bone mineral density and reduce the incidence of vertebral fractures.

**ACTION/KINETICS:** Inhibits osteoclast activity and reduces bone resorption and turnover. In postmenopausal women, the drug reduces the elevated rate of bone turnover, leading to a net gain in bone mass. **Time to maximum plasma levels, after PO:** 0.5–2 hr. Absorption is impaired by food or beverages (other than plain water). After absorption, ibandronate either binds rapidly to bone or is excreted in the urine. Drug not bound to bone is excreted unchanged by the kidney (about 50–60% of the absorbed dose). Unabsorbed drug is excreted unchanged in the feces. **$t\frac{1}{2}$, terminal, after PO:** 10–60 hr.

**SIDE EFFECTS:** Back/arm/leg pain, diarrhea, dyspepsia, abdominal pain, constipation, pain/difficulty swallowing, headache, nausea, rash.

---

**DOSAGE: IV only**

*Postmenopausal osteoporosis.*

**Adults:** 3 mg q 3 months given over 15–30 seconds.

**DOSAGE: Tablets**

*Treat or prevent postmenopausal osteoporosis.*

**Adults:** 2.5 mg once daily or one 150 mg tablet taken once monthly on the same date each month.

---

**NEED TO KNOW**

1. Do not use in clients unable to stand or sit upright for at least 60 min.

2. Use with caution with aspirin or NSAIDs.
3. Greater sensitivity can not be ruled out in some geriatric clients.
4. Therapy must include calcium and vitamin D supplements.
5. Do not mix the injection with calcium-containing solutions or other IV administered drugs.
6. If the IV dose is missed, administer as soon as it can be rescheduled. Thereafter, schedule injections every 3 months from the date of the last injection.
7. Take as directed once daily at least 60 min before the first food or drink (other than water) of the day and before any PO medications containing Al, calcium, or Mg, including supplements and vitamins.
8. If once-monthly dose is missed, and the next scheduled ibandronate day is more than 7 days away, take one 150 mg tablet in the morning of the date that it is remembered. Return to taking the one 150 mg tablet every month in the morning of the chosen day, according to the original schedule.
9. Swallow tablets whole with a full glass of plain water (6–8 oz) while standing or sitting in an upright position. Do not lie down for 60 min after taking the drug. Do not double up or take dose later in the day.
10. Do not take any OTC medications, vitamins, or supplements without approval; may inhibit drug action. Should be prescribed supplemental calcium and vitamin D.

## Lansoprazole    B
(lan-**SAHP**-rah-zohl)
**Rx:** Prevacid, Prevacid IV.

**CLASSIFICATION(S):** Proton pump inhibitor
**USES: PO.** (1) Short-term treatment (up to 4 weeks) for healing and symptomatic relief of active duodenal ulcer (PO only). (2) Maintain healing of duodenal ulcer (PO only). (3) With clarithro-

mycin and/or amoxicillin to eradicate *Helicobacter pylori* infection in active or recurrent duodenal ulcers (PO only). (4) Short-term treatment (up to 8 weeks) for healing and symptomatic relief of active benign gastric ulcer. (5) Treatment of NSAID-associated gastric ulcer in those who continue NSAID use. (6) Reduce the risk of NSAID-associated gastric ulcer in those with a history of documented gastric ulcer who required an NSAID (PO only). (7) Short-term treatment (up to 8 weeks) for healing and symptomatic relief of all grades of erosive esophagitis. Maintain healing of erosive esophagitis. (8) Long-term treatment of pathologic hypersecretory conditions, including Zollinger-Ellison syndrome (PO only). (9) Heartburn and other symptoms of GERD. (10) Short-term treatment of symptomatic GERD and erosive esophagitis. **IV.** Short-term (up to 7 days) treatment of all grades of erosive esophagitis. Then, switch to PO lansoprazole formulations.

**ACTION/KINETICS:** Drug is a gastric acid (proton) pump inhibitor in that it blocks the final step of acid production. Suppresses gastric acid secretion by inhibition of the $(H^+, K^+)$-ATPase system located at the secretory surface of the parietal cells in the stomach. Both basal and stimulated gastric acid secretion are inhibited, regardless of the stimulus. May have antimicrobial activity against *H. pylori*. Absorption begins only after lansoprazole granules leave the stomach, but absorption is rapid. Bioavailability is greater than 80%. **Peak plasma levels:** 1.7 hr. **Mean plasma $t\frac{1}{2}$, PO:** 1.5 hr; **IV:** 1.3 hr. **Onset:** 1–3 hr. **Duration:** Over 24 hr. Food does not appear to affect the rate of absorption, if given before meals. Metabolized in the liver with metabolites excreted through both the urine (33%) and feces (66%).

**SIDE EFFECTS:** Diarrhea, headache, N&V, constipation, rash. *GI HEMORRHAGE, RECTAL HEMORRHAGE, PANCREATITIS, CVA, MI, SHOCK, PANCYTOPENIA, APLASTIC ANEMIA, STEVENS-JOHNSON SYNDROME, TOXIC EPIDERMAL NECROLYSIS, ALLERGIC REACTION, ANAPHYLACTOID-LIKE REACTION.*

**DOSAGE: Capsules, Delayed-Release; Oral Suspension, Delayed-Release; Tablets, Orally Disintegrating, Delayed-Release**

*Treatment of duodenal ulcer.*

    **Adults, short-term treatment:** 15 mg once daily before breakfast for 4 weeks.

*Maintenance of healed duodenal ulcer.*

    **Adults:** 15 mg once daily.

*Duodenal ulcer associated with H. pylori infections.*

    **Adults:** The following regimens may be used: (1) *Triple therapy.* Lansoprazole, 30 mg, plus clarithromycin, 500 mg, plus amoxicillin, 1 gram, each taken twice a day (q 12 hr) for 10 or 14 days. (2) *Dual Therapy.* Lansoprazole, 30 mg plus amoxicillin, 1 gram each taken 3 times per day (q 8 hr) for 14 days (for clients intolerant or resistant to clarithromycin).

*Treatment of gastric ulcer.*

    **Adults:** 30 mg once daily for up to 8 weeks.

*Reduce risk of NSAID-associated gastric ulcer.*

    **Adults:** 15 mg once daily for up to 12 weeks.

*Treatment of NSAID-associated gastric ulcer.*

    **Adults:** 30 mg once daily for 8 weeks.

*GERD.*

    **Adults:** 15 mg once daily for up to 8 weeks.

*Erosive esophagitis.*

    **Adults, short-term treatment:** 30 mg once daily before meals for up to 8 weeks. For adults who do not heal in 8 weeks, an additional 8 weeks of therapy may be given. If there is a recurrence, an additional 8-week course may be considered. **Maintenance:** 15 mg once daily.

*Pathologic hypersecretory conditions (including Zollinger-Ellison syndrome).*

    **Adults:** Individualize dose. **Initial:** 60 mg once daily. Adjust

the dose to client need. Dosage may be continued as long as
necessary. Doses up to 90 or 120 mg (in divided doses) daily
have been given. Some clients have been treated for longer
than 4 years.

## DOSAGE: IV

*Erosive esophagitis.*
**Adults:** 30 mg/day given over 30 min for up to 7 days. When
able to take PO medication, switch to PO Prevacid and continue for up to 6–8 weeks.

## NEED TO KNOW

1. Symptomatic relief does not preclude the presence of gastric
   malignancy.
2. Do not crush or chew any lansoprazole PO product.
3. For those unable to swallow capsules, open delayed-release
   capsule and sprinkle contents on a tablespoon of applesauce,
   *Ensure,* pudding, cottage cheese, yogurt, or strained pears and
   swallow immediately. Alternatively, contents of the capsule
   can be mixed with about 2 oz of either apple, orange, or to-
   mato juice, mixed briefly, and swallowed immediately. To ensure complete delivery of the medication, rinse the glass with
   2 or more volumes of juice and swallow contents immediately. Do not chew or crush the granules.
4. The delayed-release, orally disintegrating tablets may be giv-
   en with an oral syringe or NG tube. To give via syringe or NG
   tube, dissolve a 15 mg tablet in 4 mL water or a 30 mg tablet
   in 10 mL water; shake gently and give within 15 min. Refill the
   syringe with approximately 5 mL of water, shake gently, and
   flush the NG tube.
5. Take as prescribed (usually 30 min before meals); do not exceed dose or share medications. Place orally disintegrating
   tablets on the tongue and allow to dissolve and then swallow
   small particles.
6. May have to stop drug if reports of any severe headaches,
   worsening of symptoms, fever, chills, or diarrhea.

7. Avoid hazardous activities until drug effects realized; dizziness may occur.
8. Avoid alcohol, aspirin, NSAIDs, and OTC agents unless prescribed; may increase GI irritation.

## Latanoprost
(lah-**TAH**-noh-prost)
**Rx:** Xalatan.

**C**

**CLASSIFICATION(S):** Prostaglandin agonist
**USES:** Reduce intraocular pressure (IOP) in open-angle glaucoma and ocular hypertension in clients who are intolerant of other IOP lowering medications or who failed to achieve target IOP over time.
**ACTION/KINETICS:** A prostaglandin $F^2\alpha$ analog that decreases IOP by increasing the outflow of aqueous humor. Absorbed through the cornea where it is hydrolyzed by esterases to the active acid. **Peak levels in aqueous humor:** 2 hr. **Onset:** 3–4 hr. **Maximum effect:** 8–12 hr. The active acid is metabolized in the liver and excreted in the urine. **t½, elimination:** 17 min.
**SIDE EFFECTS:** Blurred vision, burning, stinging, conjunctival hyperemia, foreign body sensation, itching, increased pigmentation of the iris, punctate epithelial keratopathy.

**DOSAGE: Solution, 0.005%**
*Elevated intraocular pressure.*
   **Adults:** 1 gtt (1.5 mcg) in the affected eye(s) once daily in the evening. More frequent use may decrease the IOP lowering effect.

**NEED TO KNOW**
1. Do not use while wearing contact lenses or in active intraocular inflammation.
2. May gradually change eye color by increasing the amount of

brown pigment in the iris; the resultant color changes may be permanent.
3. May be used concomitantly with other topical ophthalmic drugs to lower IOP. If more than one drug is used, give at least 5 min apart.
4. Wash hands before and after use. Avoid touching any part of the eye with the container tip to prevent contamination and eye infections. Contaminated solutions may cause eye damage and loss of vision.

## Leflunomide
(leh-**FLOON**-oh-myd)                                          X
**Rx: Arava.**

**CLASSIFICATION(S):** Antiarthritic
**USES:** (1) Treatment of active rheumatoid arthritis in adults, including to retard structural damage. (2) Improvement of physical function in adults with active rheumatoid arthritis.
**ACTION/KINETICS:** Inhibits dihydroorotate dehydrogenase, an enzyme involved in de novo pyrimidine synthesis; has antiproliferative activity and anti-inflammatory and uricosuric effects. After PO, is metabolized to an active metabolite (M1). **Peak levels, M1:** 6–12 hr. **t½, M1:** About 2 weeks. M1 is extensively bound to albumin. M1 is further metabolized and excreted through the kidney (more significant over the first 96 hr) and bile.
**SIDE EFFECTS:** Diarrhea, respiratory infection, hypertension, alopecia, rash, headache, nausea, bronchitis, dyspepsia, GI/abdominal pain, back pain, UTI. *HEPATIC NECROSIS, SERIOUS HEPATIC INJURY.*

## DOSAGE: Tablets
*Rheumatoid arthritis.*
> **Adults, loading dose:** 100 mg/day PO for 3 days. **Maintenance:** 20 mg/day; if this dose is not well tolerated, decrease to 10 mg/day. Doses greater than 20 mg/day are not recommended due to increased risk of side effects.

**NEED TO KNOW**

1. Do not use in hepatic insufficiency, or positive hepatitis B or C. Also, do not use in those with severe immunodeficiency, bone marrow dysplasia, severe uncontrolled infections, or vaccination with live vaccines.

2. Clients have died from interstitial lung disease that developed during therapy; onset or worsening of cough or dyspnea may require further evaluation; the drug elimination process may be required.

3. Aspirin, NSAIDs, or low-dose corticosteroids may be continued during leflunomide therapy.

4. Use the drug elimination procedure to achieve nondetectable plasma levels (less than 0.02 mcg/mL) after stopping treatment: Give cholestyramine, 8 grams 3 times per day for 11 days (no need to be consecutive unless need to lower plasma levels rapidly). Verify plasma levels by two separate tests at least 14 days apart. Without the drug elimination procedure, it may take 2 years or less to reach plasma M1 levels of 0.02 mcg/mL due to variations in drug clearance.

5. May take with or without food; takes up to 8 weeks for desired effects.

6. May experience dizziness, diarrhea, nausea, GI upset, URI, headache, and rash; report if persistent or intolerable.

---

## Levodopa
(lee-voh-**DOH**-pah)
**Rx:** Dopar, L-Dopa, Larodopa.

**CLASSIFICATION(S):** Antiparkinson drug
**USES:** Idiopathic, arteriosclerotic, or postencephalitic parkinsonism due to carbon monoxide or manganese intoxication and in the elderly associated with cerebral arteriosclerosis. Levodopa only provides symptomatic relief and does not alter the course of

the disease. When effective, it relieves rigidity, bradykinesia, tremors, dysphagia, seborrhea, sialorrhea, and postural instability.
**ACTION/KINETICS:** Depletion of dopamine in the striatum of the brain is thought to cause the symptoms of Parkinson's disease. Levodopa, a dopamine precursor, is able to cross the blood-brain barrier to enter the CNS. It is decarboxylated to dopamine in the basal ganglia, thus replenishing depleted dopamine stores. **Peak plasma levels:** 0.5–2 hr (may be delayed if ingested with food). $t^{1/2}$, **plasma:** 1–3 hr. **Onset:** 2–3 weeks, although some clients may require up to 6 months. Extensively metabolized (more than 95%) both in the periphery and the liver; metabolites are excreted in the urine.
**SIDE EFFECTS:** Choreiform and/or dystonic movements, anorexia, N&V, abdominal pain, dry mouth, dysphagia, dysgeusia, headache, dizziness, sialorrhea, malaise, fatigue, euphoria. The side effects of levodopa are numerous and usually dose related. *SEIZURES, HEMOLYTIC ANEMIA, AGRANULOCYTOSIS.*

---

**DOSAGE: Capsules; Tablets**
*Parkinsonism.*
> **Adults, initial:** 250 mg 2–4 times per day taken with food; **then,** increase total daily dose by no more than 750 mg/day q 3–7 days until optimum dosage reached (should not exceed 8 grams/day). Up to 6 months may be required to achieve a significant therapeutic effect.

---

**NEED TO KNOW**
1. Do not use with MAOIs, except MAO-B inhibitors (e.g., selegiline).
2. Use with extreme caution in clients with history of MIs, convulsions, arrhythmias, bronchial asthma, emphysema, active peptic ulcer, psychosis or neurosis, wide-angle glaucoma, and renal, hepatic, or endocrine diseases.
3. Geriatric clients may require a lower dose as they have a reduced tolerance for the drug and its side effects (including cardiac effects).

4. If unable to swallow tablets or capsules, crush tablets or empty the capsule into a small amount of fruit juice at the time of administration.

5. Often administered together with an anticholinergic agent.

6. Take exactly as prescribed; may take with food to decrease GI upset.

7. Report headaches; may indicate drug-induced glaucoma. Twitching or eye spasms may indicate toxicity.

8. Avoid fortified cereals and taking multivitamin preparations containing 10–25 mg of $B_6$ as they may reverse the antiparkinson effect.

9. May cause dizziness or drowsiness. Do not perform tasks that require mental alertness until drug effects realized. Change from a sitting or lying position slowly, and wear elastic hose to decrease dizziness.

10. Report any evidence of depression or psychosis, or other unusual mental or behavioral changes.

---

## Levothyroxine sodium ($T_4$) ■ A
(lee-voh-thigh-**ROX**-een)

**Rx:** Levothroid, Levoxyl, Synthroid, Thyro-Tabs, Tirosint, Unithroid.

**CLASSIFICATION(S):** Thyroid product

**USES:** (1) Replacement or supplemental therapy for congenital or acquired hypothyroidism of any etiology, except transient hypothyroidism during the recovery phase of subacute thyroiditis. (2) Treatment or prevention of various types of euthyroid goiters, including thyroid nodules, subacute or chronic lymphocytic thyroiditis, and multinodular goiter. (3) Adjunct to surgery and radioiodine therapy to manage thyrotropin-dependent well-differentiated thyroid cancer.

**ACTION/KINETICS:** Levothyroxine is the synthetic sodium salt of the levoisomer of $T_4$ (tetraiodothyronine). Levothyroxine, 50–60

mcg equals approximately 60 mg (1 grain) of thyroid. Absorption from the GI tract is incomplete and variable, especially when taken with food. Has a slower onset but a longer duration than sodium liothyronine. More active on a weight basis than thyroid. Is usually the drug of choice. Effect is predictable as thyroid content is standard. **Time to peak therapeutic effect:** 3–4 weeks. **t½:** 6–7 days in a euthyroid person, 9–10 days in a hypothyroid client, and 3–4 days in a hyperthyroid client. **Duration:** 1–3 weeks after withdrawal of chronic therapy. *NOTE:* All levothyroxine products are not bioequivalent; thus, changing brands is not recommended.
**SIDE EFFECTS:** Symptoms of hyperthyroidism.

## DOSAGE: Capsules; Tablets

*Mild hypothyroidism.*
> **Adults, initial:** 50 mcg once daily; **then,** increase by 25–50 mcg q 2–3 weeks until desired clinical response is attained. **Maintenance, usual:** 75–125 mcg/day (although doses up to 200 mcg/day may be required in some clients).

*Severe hypothyroidism.*
> **Adults, initial:** 12.5–25 mcg once daily; **then,** increase dose, as necessary, in increments of 25 mcg at 2- to 3-week intervals.

## DOSAGE: IM; IV

*Myxedematous coma.*
> **Adults, initial:** 400 mcg by rapid IV injection, even in geriatric clients; **then,** 100–200 mcg/day, IV. **Maintenance:** 100–200 mcg/day, IV. Smaller daily doses should be given until client can tolerate PO medication.

*Hypothyroidism.*
> **Adults:** 50–100 mcg once daily.

*TSH suppression in well-differentiated thyroid cancer or thyroid nodules.*
> **Adults:** Individualize dose. **Usual dose:** 2 mcg/kg/day.

## NEED TO KNOW

1. In euthyroid clients, doses within the range of daily hormonal

requirements are ineffective for weight reduction. Larger doses may produce serious or even life-threatening manifestations of toxicity, especially when given with sympathomimetic amines such as those used for their anorectic effects.

2. Errors have occurred when prescribers have ordered 0.25 mg (250 mcg) instead of the correct dose of 0.025 mg (25 mcg). Be careful with decimal point placements and when converting a dose from micrograms to milligrams.

3. Take with a full glass of water to prevent choking, gagging, dysphagia, or getting tablets stuck in the throat.

4. Transfer from liothyronine to levothyroxine: Administer replacement drug for several days before discontinuing liothyronine. Transfer from levothyroxine to liothyronine: Discontinue levothyroxine before starting low daily dose of liothyronine.

5. Take at the same time each day on an empty stomach 1 hr before or 2–3 hr after a meal. Take in the morning to prevent insomnia. Do not take with food unless specifically instructed; may interfere with absorption. Avoid iodine-rich foods.

6. Report severe headache, palpitations, chest pain, diarrhea, irritability, excitability, insomnia, intolerance to heat, significant weight loss, and/or excessive sweating.

7. If taking raloxifene, take levothyroxine at least 12 hr earlier in the day.

## Lorazepam     D
(lor-**AYZ**-eh-pam)
**Rx:** Ativan, Lorazepam Intensol, **C-IV.**

**CLASSIFICATION(S):** Antianxiety drug, benzodiazepine
**USES: PO:** Short-term relief of anxiety disorders or symptoms of anxiety with depression. **Parenteral:** (1) Preanesthetic medication to produce sedation, relief of anxiety, and a decreased ability to recall events related to surgery. (2) Status epilepticus.

**ACTION/KINETICS:** Reduces anxiety by increasing or facilitating the inhibitory neurotransmitter activity of GABA. Absorbed and eliminated faster than other benzodiazepines. **Peak plasma levels, PO:** 1–6 hr; **IM:** 1–1.5 hr. **t½:** 10–20 hr. Metabolized to inactive compounds, which are excreted through the kidneys.

**SIDE EFFECTS:** Drowsiness (transient), ataxia, confusion.

## DOSAGE: Oral Concentrate; Tablets

*Anxiety.*

**Adults, initial:** 2–3 mg/day given 2 or 3 times per day. Dose range varies from 1 to 10 mg/day given in divided doses.

*Insomnia due to anxiety or transient situational stress.*

**Adults:** Single dose of 2–4 mg at bedtime.

## DOSAGE: IM

*Preanesthetic.*

**Adults:** 0.05 mg/kg, up to a maximum of 4 mg. For optimum effect, give at least 2 hr before surgical procedure. Administer narcotic analgesics at their usual preoperative time.

## DOSAGE: IV

*Status epilepticus.*

**Adults, usual:** 4 mg given slowly (2 mg/min). If seizures continue or recur after a 10–15-min period, an additional 4 mg IV may be given slowly.

*Preanesthetic.*

**Adults, initial:** 2 mg total or 0.044 mg/kg (whichever is smaller). This will sedate most adults. Do not exceed dose in clients over 50 years of age. Doses as high as 0.05 mg/kg (up to a total of 4 mg) may be given if a greater lack of recall is desired. For optimum effect, give 15–20 min prior to procedure.

## NEED TO KNOW

1. For the elderly or debilitated, start with 1–2 mg/day of tablet or solution in divided doses. Adjust dose as needed and tolerated. When higher doses are needed, increase the evening dose before the daytime dose.

2. Intensol product is a concentrated PO solution. Mix with liquid or semi-solid foods such as water, juices, soda or soda-like beverages, applesauce, or puddings.

3. IM administration is not recommended for status epilepticus as therapeutic levels may not be reached as quickly as with IV. IM can be used when an IV port is not available.

4. Reduce dose of lorazepam by 50% when given with probenecid or valproate.

5. For IV use, dilute just before use with equal amounts of either sterile water, NaCl, or 5% dextrose injection. Do not shake vigorously; will result in air entrapment.

6. Inject directly into tubing of an existing IV infusion. Do not exceed 2 mg/min IV. Have available equipment to maintain a patent airway.

7. May cause dizziness, drowsiness, loss of recall; use with caution until drug effects realized.

8. Avoid alcohol and CNS depressants.

## Lovastatin (Mevinolin)
**(LOW-**vah-**STAT-**in, me-**VIN-**oh-lin)
**Rx:** Altoprev, Mevacor.

**CLASSIFICATION(S):** Antihyperlipidemic, HMG-CoA reductase inhibitor

**USES: Immediate-Release Only:** As an adjunct to diet to reduce elevated total and LDL cholesterol in primary hypercholesterolemia (types IIa and IIb) when the response to diet restricted in saturated fat and cholesterol and to other nonpharmacological regimens has been inadequate. **Extended-Release Only:** Adjunct to diet to decrease elevated total and LDL cholesterol, Apo B, and triglycerides and to increase HDL cholesterol in those with primary hypercholesterolemia (heterozygous familial and nonfamilial and mixed dyslipidemia Fredrickson types IIa and IIb) when response to diet restricted in saturated fat and cholesterol and other nonpharmacological measures have been inadequate. **Immediate-Release or Extended-Release:** (1) To slow the progression of coronary atherosclerosis in clients with CAD in order to lower total and LDL cholesterol levels to target levels. (2) Primary prevention of coronary heart disease in those without symptomatic CV disease, average to moderately elevated total cholesterol and LDL cholesterol, and below average HDL cholesterol. Used to reduce risk of MI, unstable angina, and coronary revascularization procedures.

ACTION/KINETICS: Competitively inhibits HMG-CoA reductase; this enzyme catalyzes the early rate-limiting step in the synthesis of cholesterol. Thus, cholesterol synthesis is inhibited/decreased. Decreases total cholesterol, triglycerides, LDL, and VLDL and increases HDL. Extensive first-pass metabolism (by CYP2C9); less than 5% reaches the general circulation. Absorption is decreased by about one-third if the drug is given on an empty stomach rather than with food. **Onset:** Within 2 weeks using multiple doses. **Time to peak plasma levels:** 2–4 hr. **Time to peak effect:** 4–6 weeks using multiple doses. $t\frac{1}{2}$: 3–4 hr for immediate-release. **Duration:** 4–6 weeks after termination of therapy. Metabolized in the liver (its main site of action) to active metabolites. Severe renal impairment increases plasma levels. Over 80% of a PO dose is excreted in the feces, via the bile, and approximately 10% is excreted through the urine.

SIDE EFFECTS: Headache, diarrhea, flatulence, N&V, abdominal pain/cramps, constipation, dyspepsia, myalgia, back pain, rash/pruritus, flu syndrome, infection, pain.

---

DOSAGE: Tablets, Extended-Release

*Hyperlipidemia, coronary heart disease, primary prevention of coronary heart disease.*

**Adults, initial:** 20, 40, or 60 mg once a day at bedtime; **range:** 10–60 mg/day in single doses. Start with 10 mg once a day for those requiring small reductions in lipid levels. Adjust dose at intervals of 4 weeks or more.

## DOSAGE: Tablets, Immediate-Release

*Hypercholesterolemia, coronary heart disease, primary prevention of coronary heart disease.*

**Adults, initial:** 20 mg once daily with the evening meal. Initiate at 10 mg/day in clients who require smaller reductions. Initiate at 20 mg/day in those requiring reductions in LDL-C of 20% or more. **Dose range:** 10–80 mg (maximum)/day in single or two divided doses. Adjust dose at intervals of every 4 weeks, if necessary. If $C_{CR}$ is less than 30 mL/min, use doses greater than 20 mg/day with caution.

## NEED TO KNOW

1. Immediate-release is effective alone or when used together with bile acid sequestrants. Avoid use of extended-release with fibrates or niacin; if such combinations are used, do not exceed a dose of 20 mg/day of lovastatin.
2. Do not exceed dose of 40 mg/day of lovastatin if taking amiodarone or verapamil. Do not exceed a dose of 20 mg/day of lovastatin if taking cyclosporine related to increased risk of myopathy.
3. Take with meals. Avoid coadministration with grapefruit juice due to increased serum levels of lovastatin. Continue cholesterol-lowering diet and exercise program. Cholesterol production by the liver is highest in the evening; medication usually taken with the evening meal.
4. Follow a standard cholesterol-lowering diet before starting lovastatin and continue during therapy.
5. Report malaise, myalgia, muscle spasms, or fever. These may be mistaken for the flu, but could be serious side effects of drug therapy.
6. Any right upper quadrant abdominal pain or yellowing of eyes, skin, stools should be reported.
7. Periodic liver function tests and eye exams are mandatory; report early visual disturbances.

**CLASSIFICATION(S):** Drug for chronic idiopathic constipation

**USES:** Treatment of chronic idiopathic constipation in adults.

**ACTION/KINETICS:** Lubiprostone is a locally acting chloride channel activator that enhances a chloride-rich intestinal fluid secretion without changing sodium and potassium serum levels. By increasing intestinal fluid secretion the drug increases intestinal motility, thereby increasing the passage of stool and alleviating symptoms associated with chronic idiopathic constipation. The main site of action appears to be the luminal portion of the GI epithelium. Rapidly and extensively metabolized in the liver by carbonyl reductase. Excreted in the urine (60%) and feces (30%). **t½:** 0.9–1.4 hr.

**SIDE EFFECTS:** Fatigue, dizziness, headache, hypesthesia, abdominal discomfort/pain, diarrhea, flatulence, N&V, UTI, back pain, retching, dyspnea, sinusitis, URTI, chest discomfort, peripheral edema.

---

**DOSAGE: Capsules**

*Chronic idiopathic constipation.*

  **Adults:** 24 mcg twice a day with food. Periodically assess the need for continued therapy.

---

**NEED TO KNOW**

1. Do not use in those with a history of mechanical GI obstruction.
2. Take as directed with food; do not double up if dose missed.
3. May cause dizziness. Do not drive or perform activities that require mental alertness until drug effects realized. Using lubiprostone alone, with certain other medicines, or with alcohol may lessen ability to drive or perform other potentially dangerous tasks.
4. Back pain, diarrhea, dizziness, gas, heartburn, headache, nau-

sea and/or vomiting, stomach pain/upset, bloating, or tiredness may occur; report if bothersome.

**CLASSIFICATION(S):** Drug for Alzheimer's disease

**USES:** Moderate to severe dementia of the Alzheimer's type. When combined with donepezil (Aricept), the decline of mental and physical function may be less.

**ACTION/KINETICS:** It is believed that activation of N-methyl-D-aspartate (NMDA) receptors, in the brain by glutamate, an excitatory amino acid, contributes to the symptomatology of Alzheimer's disease. Memantine is believed to have low to moderate affinity as an antagonist for open-channel NMDA receptors, thus preventing activation by glutamate. The drug does not prevent or slow neurodegeneration in Alzheimer's disease. Well absorbed after PO administration; **peak levels:** 3–7 hr. Food has no effect on the absorption. Excreted mainly unchanged in the urine. **t½, terminal:** 60–80 hr.

**SIDE EFFECTS:** Fatigue, pain, increased BP, dizziness, headache, constipation, vomiting, back pain, confusion, somnolence, hallucinations, coughing, dyspnea. *GI HEMORRHAGE, CONVULSIONS, CEREBRAL HEMORRHAGE, SUICIDE ATTEMPT, CVA, CARDIAC FAILURE, MI, CARDIAC ARREST, PULMONARY EMBOLISM.*

---

**DOSAGE: Oral Solution; Tablets**

*Alzheimer's disease.*

  **Adults, initial:** 5 mg/day. Dose should be increased in 5 mg increments to 10 mg/day (5 mg twice a day), then 15 mg/day (5 mg and 10 mg as separate doses), and finally 20 mg/day (10 mg twice a day). The minimum recommended interval between dose increases is one week. Reduce the dose in clients with moderate renal impairment.

---

**NEED TO KNOW**

1. Conditions that raise urine pH may decrease the urinary elimination of memantine, resulting in increased plasma levels.

2. It is likely that clients with moderate to severe renal impairment will have higher levels of the drug; dose reduction should be considered. Use with caution in renal tubular acidosis, severe UTIs.
3. May take with or without food; with food if GI upset.
4. Avoid alcohol and any OTC products or herbals without provider approval to prevent interactions. May cause dizziness, constipation, headache, pain.

## Metformin hydrochloride    B
(met-**FOR**-min)

**Rx:** Fortamet, Glucophage, Glucophage XR, Glumetza, Riomet.

**CLASSIFICATION(S):** Antidiabetic, oral; biguanide
**USES:** (1) As monotherapy, as an adjunct to diet and exercise, to improve glycemic control in clients with non-insulin-dependent diabetes mellitus (type 2 diabetes). The immediate-release tablets and PO solution can be used in clients 10 years of age and older. (2) Extended-release form used to treat type 2 diabetes as initial therapy or in combination with a sulfonylurea or insulin in clients aged 17 years and older.
**ACTION/KINETICS:** Decreases hepatic glucose production, decreases intestinal absorption of glucose, and increases peripheral uptake and utilization of glucose. Does not cause hypoglycemia in either diabetic or nondiabetic clients, and it does not cause hyperinsulinemia. Insulin secretion remains unchanged, while fasting insulin levels and day-long plasma insulin response may decrease. Food decreases and slightly delays the absorption of metformin. Steady-state plasma levels (less than 1 mcg/mL) are reached within 24–48 hr. Excreted unchanged in the urine. **t½, plasma elimination:** 6.2 hr. The plasma and blood half-lives are prolonged with decreased renal function and in the elderly.

**SIDE EFFECTS:** Hypoglycemia, diarrhea, N&V, asthenia, flatulence, headache, abdominal pain/discomfort.

---

**DOSAGE: Oral Solution**

*Type 2 diabetes.*

 **Adults:** Individualize dosage. Up to 2,550 mg/day.

**DOSAGE: Tablets; Tablets, Extended-Release**

*Type 2 diabetes.*

 **Adults, individualize dosage regimen: Using 500-mg immediate-release tablet:** Starting dose is one 500-mg tablet twice a day given with the morning and evening meals. Dosage increases may be made in increments of 500 mg every week, given in divided doses, up to a maximum of 2,500 mg/day. If a 2,500-mg daily dose is required, it may be better tolerated when given in divided doses 3 times per day with meals. The extended-release tablet is given once daily. **Using 850-mg immediate-release tablet:** Starting dose is 850 mg once daily given with the morning meal. Dosage increases may be made in increments of 850 mg every other week, given in divided doses, up to a maximum of 2,550 mg/day. **Usual maintenance dose:** 850 mg twice a day with the morning and evening meals. However, some may require 850 mg 3 times per day with meals. **Using 500-mg extended-release tablet, Initial:** 500 mg once daily with the evening meal. Adjust dose, if needed, in increments of 500 mg/week, up to a maximum of 2,000 mg once daily with the evening meal. If glycemic control is not achieved on 2,000 mg once daily, consider 1,000 mg twice a day. If higher doses are needed, use total daily dose up to 2,550 mg given in divided doses. **Using 1,000-mg extended-release tablet: Initial:** 1,000 mg once daily with the evening meal. Dosage may be increased weekly in 500 mg increments, based on efficacy and tolerance, but must not exceed 2,500 mg/day.

---

**NEED TO KNOW**

1. Lactic acidosis is a rare, but serious, metabolic complication

that can occur due to metformin accumulation during treatment with metformin.

2. Do not use in renal disease or dysfunction (serum creatinine levels greater than 1.5 mg/dL in males and greater than 1.4 mg/dL in females) or abnormal $C_{CR}$ due to cardiovascular collapse, acute MI, or septicemia. Do not use in CHF requiring pharmacologic intervention.

3. Do not use in acute or chronic metabolic acidosis, including diabetic ketoacidosis, with or without coma.

4. Use of oral hypoglycemic agents may increase the risk of cardiovascular mortality.

5. Although hypoglycemia does not usually occur with metformin, it may result with deficient caloric intake, with strenuous exercise not supplemented by increased intake of calories, or when metformin is taken with sulfonylureas or alcohol.

6. Give with meals starting at a low dose with gradual escalation. This will reduce GI side effects and allow determination of the minimal dose necessary for adequate blood sugar control.

7. If maximum dose of metformin for 4 weeks does not provide adequate control of blood glucose, gradual addition of an oral sulfonylurea (data are available for glyburide, chlorpropamide, tolbutamide, and glipizide) may be considered, while maintaining maximum dose of metformin. Desired control of blood glucose may be attained by adjusting the dose of each drug.

8. Be conservative with initial and maintenance doses in the elderly because of possible decreased renal function. Generally, do not titrate geriatric clients to the maximum dose. Do not start metformin or metformin extended-release in clients 80 years and older unless tests show renal function is not decreased.

9. Take with food to decrease GI upset. Do not crush or chew extended-release tablets.

10. May cause a metallic taste; should subside.

11. Avoid alcohol and situations that may precipitate dehydration.

12. Stop drug and immediately report any symptoms of difficulty

breathing, severe weakness, muscle pain, increased sleepiness, dizziness, palpitation, or sudden increased abdominal distress.

# Metoclopramide

(meh-toe-kloh-**PRAH**-myd)

**B**

**Rx:** Maxolon, Reglan.

**CLASSIFICATION(S):** Gastrointestinal stimulant

**USES: PO:** (1) Short-term (4 to 12 weeks) therapy for adults with symptomatic documented gastroesophageal reflux who fail to respond to conventional treatment. (2) Symptomatic relief of acute and recurrent diabetic gastroparesis. Relief of vomiting and anorexia may precede the relief of abdominal fullness by 1 week or more. **Parenteral:** (1) Prevention of N&V associated with emetogenic cancer chemotherapy. (2) Prevention of postoperative N&V when nasogastric suction is undesirable. (3) Facilitate small bowel intubation when the tube does not pass the pylorus with conventional methods (use single doses). (4) Stimulate gastric emptying and intestinal transit of barium in clients where delayed emptying interferes with radiological examination of the stomach or small intestine. (5) Symptomatic relief of diabetic gastroparesis.

**ACTION/KINETICS:** Dopamine antagonist that acts by increasing sensitivity to acetylcholine; results in increased motility of the upper GI tract and relaxation of the pyloric sphincter and duodenal bulb. Gastric emptying time and GI transit time are shortened. Facilitates intubation of the small bowel and speeds transit of a barium meal. **Onset, IV:** 1–3 min; **IM:** 10–15 min; **PO:** 30–60 min. **Duration:** 1–2 hr. **t½:** 5–6 hr. Significant first-pass effect following PO use; unchanged drug and metabolites excreted in urine. Renal impairment decreases clearance of the drug.

**SIDE EFFECTS:** Extrapyramidal symptoms, restlessness, drowsiness, fatigue, lassitude, akathisia, dizziness, nausea, diarrhea. *DEPRESSION (WITH SUICIDAL IDEATION), SEIZURES, ANGRANULOCYTOSIS, HYPERTHERMIA.*

## DOSAGE: Syrup; Tablets

*Diabetic gastroparesis.*

**Adults:** 10 mg 30 min before meals and at bedtime for 2–8 weeks (therapy should be reinstituted if symptoms recur).

*Gastroesophageal reflux.*

**Adults:** 10–15 mg 4 times per day, 30 min before meals and at bedtime. If symptoms occur only intermittently, single doses up to 20 mg prior to the provoking situation may be used.

*Postoperative gastric bezoars.*

**Adults:** 10 mg 3–4 times per day.

## DOSAGE: IM; IV

*Diabetic gastroparesis.*

**Adults:** 10 mg 30 min before each meal and at bedtime for 2–8 weeks. May take up to 10 days for symptoms to subside; then, begin PO therapy. Reinstitute therapy at the earliest manifestation.

*Prophylaxis of vomiting due to chemotherapy.*

**Adults, initial:** 2 mg/kg IV (1 mg/kg may be adequate for less emetogenic regimens) q 2 hr for two doses, with the first dose 30 min before chemotherapy; **then,** 10 mg or more q 3 hr for three doses. Inject slowly IV over 15 min.

*Prophylaxis of postoperative N&V.*

**Adults:** 10–20 mg IM near the end of surgery.

*Facilitate small bowel intubation.*

**Adults, IV:** 10 mg.

*Radiologic examinations to increase intestinal transit time.*

**Adults:** 10 mg as a single dose given IV over 1–2 min.

## NEED TO KNOW

1. Do not use in gastrointestinal hemorrhage, obstruction, or perforation; epilepsy; clients taking drugs likely to cause extrapyramidal symptoms, such as phenothiazines.

2. Extrapyramidal effects are more likely to occur in geriatric clients.
3. If $C_{CR}$ is less than 40 mL/min, begin therapy at approximately one-half the recommended dosage. Depending on efficacy and safety, the dose may be increased or decreased as needed.
4. After PO use, absorption of certain drugs from the GI tract may be affected.
5. Metoclopramide is physically/chemically incompatible with a number of drugs; check package insert if drug is to be admixed.
6. Take as directed; may dilute syrup in water, juice, or carbonated beverage just before taking.
7. Avoid alcohol and CNS depressants.
8. Extrapyramidal effects (trembling hands, facial grimacing) should be reported; may be treated with parenteral diphenhydramine.

---

## Metoprolol succinate
(me-toe-**PROH**-lohl)          **B,C**

**Rx:** Toprol XL.

## Metoprolol tartrate

**Rx:** Lopressor.

**CLASSIFICATION(S):** Beta-adrenergic blocking agent

**USES: Metoprolol Succinate:** (1) Alone or with other drugs to treat hypertension. (2) Chronic management of angina pectoris. (3) Treatment of stable, symptomatic (NYHA Class II or III) heart failure of ischemic, hypertensive, or cardiomyopathic origin. **Metoprolol Tartrate:** (1) Hypertension (either alone or with other antihypertensive agents, such as thiazide diuretics). (2) Acute MI in hemodynamically stable clients. (3) Angina pectoris.

**ACTION/KINETICS:** Combines reversibly mainly with beta$_1$-adrenergic receptors to block the response to sympathetic nerve impulses, circulating catecholamines, or adrenergic drugs. Blockade

of beta$_1$-receptors decreases HR, myocardial contractility, and CO and slows AV conduction, all of which lead to a decrease in BP. Beta$_2$-receptors are blocked at high doses. **Onset:** 15 min. **Peak plasma levels:** 90 min. **t½:** 3–7 hr. Effect of drug is cumulative. Food increases bioavailability. Exhibits significant first-pass effect. Metabolized in liver and excreted in urine.
**SIDE EFFECTS:** Fatigue, dizziness, depression, shortness of breath, bradycardia, diarrhea.

---

**DOSAGE: Tablets, Extended-Release** METOPROLOL SUCCINATE

*Angina pectoris.*
**Adults, individualized initial:** 100 mg/day in a single dose. Dose may be increased slowly, at weekly intervals, until optimum effect is reached or there is a pronounced slowing of HR. Doses above 400 mg/day have not been studied.

*Hypertension.*
**Adults, initial:** 25–100 mg/day in a single dose with or without a diuretic. Dosage may be increased in weekly intervals until maximum effect is reached. Doses above 400 mg/day have not been studied.

*CHF.*
**Adults, individualize, initial:** 25 mg once daily for 2 weeks in clients with NYHA Class II heart failure and 12.5 mg once daily in those with more severe heart failure. Double the dose q 2 weeks to the highest dose level tolerated or up to 200 mg.

**DOSAGE: Tablets** METOPROLOL TARTRATE

*Hypertension.*
**Adults, initial:** 100 mg/day in single or divided doses; **then,** dose may be increased weekly to maintenance level of 100–450 mg/day. A diuretic may also be used.

*Angina pectoris.*
**Adults, initial:** 100 mg/day in 2 divided doses. Dose may be increased gradually at weekly intervals until optimum response is obtained or a pronounced slowing of HR occurs. Ef-

lective dose range: 100–400 mg/day. If treatment is to be discontinued, reduce dose gradually over 1–2 weeks.

**DOSAGE: Injection (IV); Tablets**

*Early treatment of MI.*

**Adults:** Three IV bolus injections of 5 mg each at approximately 2-min intervals. If client tolerates the full IV dose, give 50 mg q 6 hr PO beginning 15 min after the last IV dose (or as soon as client's condition allows). This dose is continued for 48 hr followed by **late treatment:** 100 mg twice a day as soon as feasible; continue for 1–3 months (although data suggest treatment should be continued for 1–3 years). In clients who do not tolerate the full IV dose, begin with 25–50 mg q 6 hr PO beginning 15 min after the last IV dose or as soon as client's condition allows.

**NEED TO KNOW**

1. Do not use in clients with myocardial infarction with a HR of less than 45 bpm, in second- or third-degree heart block, or if systolic blood pressure is less than 100 mm Hg. Moderate to severe cardiac failure.
2. For CHF, do not increase dose until symptoms of worsening CHF have been stabilized. Initial difficulty with titration should not preclude attempts later to use metoprolol.
3. Take at same time each day; do not stop suddenly.
4. Take with food. Do not crush or chew the extended-release products; swallow tablets whole.
5. Report any symptoms of fluid overload such as sudden weight gain, shortness of breath, or swelling of extremities. Avoid salt.

**Mometasone furoate monohydrate** C
(moh-**MET**-ah-sohn)
**Rx:** Nasonex.
**Mometasone furoate**
**Rx: Cream, Lotion, Ointment:** Elocon. **Powder for Inhalation:** Asmanex Twisthaler.

**CLASSIFICATION(S):** Glucocorticoid
**USES: Mometasone furoate monohydrate. Spray:** (1) Treatment of the nasal symptoms of seasonal allergic rhinitis and perennial allergic rhinitis in adults. (2) Prophylaxis of nasal symptoms of seasonal or perennial allergic rhinitis in adults. (3) Treatment of nasal polyps. **Mometasone furoate. Cream, Lotion, Ointment, Topical Solution:** Dermatoses. **Powder for Inhalation:** (1) Maintenance treatment of chronic asthma. (2) For asthma clients who require PO corticosteroid therapy, where adding mometasone may reduce or eliminate the need for PO corticosteroids.
**ACTION/KINETICS:** Anti-inflammatory due to ability to inhibit prostaglandin synthesis. Also inhibits accumulation of macrophages and leukocytes at sites of inflammation as well as inhibits phagocytosis and lysosomal enzyme release. Undetected in plasma although some may be swallowed after use. No effect on adrenal function. Metabolized in the liver by CYP3A4 enzymes. **t½:** 5.8 hr. Excreted in the feces and urine.
**SIDE EFFECTS: Asmanex:** Dry/irritated throat, hoarseness, cough, dry mouth, taste alteration. **Nasonex:** Headache, pharyngitis, epistaxis, nasal burning/irritation.

**DOSAGE: Nasal Spray** MOMETASONE FUROATE MONOHYDRATE
*Prophylaxis and treatment of seasonal/perennial allergic rhinitis.*
   **Adults:** Two sprays (50 mcg in each spray) into each nostril once daily (i.e., total daily dose: 200 mcg). In those with a known seasonal allergen that precipitates seasonal allergic rhi-

fiitis, give prophylactically, 200 mcg/day, 2–4 weeks prior to the anticipated start of the pollen season.

*Treatment of nasal polyps.*

**Adults:** Two sprays (100 mcg) into each nostril twice a day (i.e., total daily dose of 400 mcg). In some, a dose of two sprays once daily into each nostril (i.e., total daily dose of 200 mcg) may be effective.

## DOSAGE: Cream, Lotion, Ointment MOMETASONE FUROATE

*Dermatoses.*

**Adults:** Apply sparingly to affected area(s) 2–4 times per day.

## DOSAGE: Topical Solution

*Dermatoses.*

**Adults:** Apply a few drops to the affected skin once a day; massage lightly until solution disappears.

## DOSAGE: Powder for Inhalation

*Chronic asthma.*

**Adults: Recommended starting dose, previous therapy of bronchodilators alone or inhaled corticosteroids:** 220 mcg once daily in the evening; **highest recommended daily dose:** 440 mcg. **Recommended starting dose, previous therapy of oral corticosteroids:** 440 mcg twice daily; **highest recommended daily dose:** 880 mcg.

---

### NEED TO KNOW

1. Do not use in those with recent nasal septum ulcers, nasal surgery, or nasal trauma until healing has occurred. Not indicated to relieve acute bronchospasms.
2. Use with caution, if at all, in clients with active or quiescent tuberculosis infection of the respiratory tract, or in untreated fungal, bacterial, systemic viral infections, or ocular herpes simplex.
3. Maximum benefit: Within 1 to 2 weeks.
4. Shake nasal spray well before using.
5. Prior to initial use, prime the pump by actuating 10 times or until a fine spray appears. If more than 1 week has elapsed be-

tween use, reprime by actuating 2 times, or until a fine spray appears.

6. Do not increase dose/frequency; does not increase effectiveness. A spacer facilitates oral inhaler administration.
7. When using oral inhaler, inhale deeply and rapidly and hold breath for about 10 seconds, or as long as possible. Do not breathe out through the inhaler. Rinse mouth/equipment after inhalation use.

## Naproxen
(nah-**PROX**-en) ■ **B**

**Rx:** EC-Naprosyn, Naprosyn.

## Naproxen sodium

**OTC:** Aleve, Midol Extended Relief. **Rx:** Anaprox, Anaprox DS, Naprelan.

**CLASSIFICATION(S):** Nonsteroidal anti-inflammatory

**USES:** *Rx.* (1) Mild to moderate pain. (2) Musculoskeletal and soft-tissue inflammation including rheumatoid arthritis, osteoarthritis, bursitis, tendonitis, ankylosing spondylitis. (3) Acute gout. *NOTE:* The delayed-release or enteric-coated products are not recommended for initial treatment of pain because, compared to other naproxen products, absorption is delayed. **OTC.** (1) Relief of minor aches and pains due to the common cold, headache, toothache, muscular aches, backache, minor arthritis pain. (2) Antipyretic.

**ACTION/KINETICS:** Anti-inflammatory effect is likely due to inhibition of cyclo-oxygenase. Inhibition of cyclo-oxygenase results in decreased prostaglandin synthesis. Effective in reducing joint swelling, pain, and morning stiffness, as well as increasing mobility in those with inflammatory disease. Does not alter the course of the disease, however. The antipyretic action occurs by decreasing prostaglandin synthesis in the hypothalamus resulting in an increase in peripheral blood flow and heat loss, as well as promoting sweating. **Peak serum levels of naproxen:** 2–4 hr; **for sodium salt:** 1–2 hr. **t½ for naproxen:** 12–15 hr; **for sodium salt:** 12–13 hr. **Onset, immediate-release for analgesia:** 1–2 hr. **Duration, analgesia:** Approximately 7 hr. **Onset (both immediate- and delayed-release):** 30 min; **duration:** 24 hr. **Onset, anti-inflammatory effects:** Up to 2 weeks; **duration:** 2–4 weeks. Food delays the rate but not the amount of drug absorbed. 95% excreted in the urine.

**SIDE EFFECTS:** Headache, dizziness, drowsiness, pruritus, skin eruptions, constipation, dyspepsia/indigestion, ecchymoses, edema, dyspnea, tinnitus.

---

**DOSAGE: Rx: Oral Suspension; Tablets; Tablets, Controlled-Release; Tablets, Delayed-Release** NAPROXEN, NAPROXEN SODIUM

*Rheumatoid arthritis, osteoarthritis, ankylosing spondylitis, pain, acute tendonitis, bursitis.*

**Adults: Naproxen Tablets:** 250–500 mg twice a day. May increase to 1.5 grams for short periods of time. **Naproxen Suspension:** 250 mg (10 mL), 375 mg (15 mL), or 500 mg (20 mL) twice a day. **Naproxen, Delayed-Release (EC-Naprosyn):** 375–500 mg twice a day. **Naproxen Sodium:** 275–500 mg twice a day. May increase to 1.65 grams/day for limited periods. **Naproxen Sodium, Controlled-Release (Naprelan):** 750 mg or 1,000 mg once daily, not to exceed 1,500 mg/day. Do not exceed 1.25 grams naproxen (1.375 grams naproxen sodium) per day. If no improvement is seen within 2 weeks, consider an additional 2-week course of therapy.

*Acute gout.*

**Adults, Naproxen, initial:** 750 mg; **then,** 250 mg q 8 hr until symptoms subside. **Naproxen Sodium, initial:** 825 mg; **then,** 275 mg q 8 hr until symptoms subside. **Naproxen Sodium, Controlled-Release (Naprelan):** 1,000–1,500 mg once daily on the first day; **then,** 1,000 mg once daily until symptoms subside.

*Mild to moderate pain, acute tendonitis, bursitis.*

**Adults: Naproxen, initial:** 500 mg; **then,** 500 mg q 12 hr or

250 mg q 6–8 hr, not to exceed 1.25 grams/day. Thereafter, do not exceed 1,000 mg/day. **Naproxen Sodium, initial:** 550 mg; **then,** 550 mg q 12 hr or 275 mg q 6–8 hr, not to
exceed 1.375 grams/day. Thereafter, do not exceed 1,100
mg/day. **Naproxen Sodium, Controlled-Release (Naprelan):**
1,000 mg once daily. For a limited time, 1,500 mg/day may be
used. Thereafter, do not exceed 1,000 mg/day.

**DOSAGE: OTC: Capsules, Liquid Gel; Tablets**

*Analgesic, antipyretic.*

**Adults:** 220 mg q 8–12 hr with a full glass of liquid. For some
clients, 440 mg initially followed by 220 mg 12 hr later will
provide better relief. Do not exceed 660 mg in a 24-hr period.
Do not exceed 220 mg q 12 hr for geriatric clients.

## NEED TO KNOW

1. NSAIDs may cause an increased risk of serious CV thrombotic
   events, MI, and stroke, which can be fatal.
2. Naproxen is contraindicated (except for controlled-released
   tablets) for treatment of perioperative pain in the setting of
   coronary artery bypass graft surgery.
3. NSAIDs cause an increased risk of serious GI adverse events including bleeding, ulceration, and perforation of the stomach
   or intestines, which can be fatal.
4. Geriatric clients may manifest increased total plasma levels of
   naproxen. Higher doses and use in those at risk of developing
   Alzheimer's disease may increase the risk of strokes and heart
   attacks.
5. To be taken in the morning and in the evening. The doses do
   not have to be equal.
6. Do not use the OTC product for more than 10 days for pain or
   3 days for fever unless prescribed.
7. Take with food and a full glass of water to reduce GI upset. Do
   not break, chew, or crush delayed-release tablets.
8. Those consuming three or more alcoholic drinks per day

should consult their provider for advice on when and how to take naproxen and other pain relievers.

9. Report lack of response, worsening of symptoms, unusual bruising/bleeding, persistent abdominal pain, sore throat, fever, rash, altered vision, joint pain, edema, or dark-colored stools. May need periodic eye exams with prolonged therapy.

10. Use protection when exposed to prolonged sunlight; may have sensitivity reaction.

---

## Nicotine polacrilex (Nicotine Resin Complex) (NIK-oh-teen)   C
**OTC:** Commit, Nicorette, Nicotine Gum.

**CLASSIFICATION(S):** Smoking deterrent
**USES:** Adjunct with behavioral modification in smokers wishing to give up the smoking habit in those 18 years and older. Is considered only as an initial aid, with the ultimate goal being abstention from all forms of nicotine.
**ACTION/KINETICS:** Following chewing, nicotine is released from an ion exchange resin in the gum product, providing blood nicotine levels approximating those produced by smoking cigarettes. The amount of nicotine released depends on the rate and duration of chewing. **Time to peak levels:** 15–30 min. **Peak plasma levels:** 5–10 ng/mL. If the gum is swallowed, only a minimum amount of nicotine is released. **t½:** 3–4 hr. Metabolized mainly by the liver, with about 10–20% excreted unchanged in the urine.
**SIDE EFFECTS:** Sore mouth/throat, nausea, salivation, dizziness.

---

**DOSAGE: Gum**

*Smoking deterrent.*

**Adults:** If the client smokes fewer than 25 cigarettes/day, start with the 2 mg nicotine gum. If the client smokes more than 25 cigarettes/day, start with the 4 mg nicotine gum. **Weeks 1–6:** 1 piece of gum q 2 hr; **Weeks 7–9:** 1 piece of gum q 2–4 hr; **Weeks 10–12:** 1 piece of gum q 4–8 hr.

M.P.

## DOSAGE: Lozenges

*Smoking deterrent.*

**Adults:** If first cigarette is smoked more than 30 min after waking, start with the 2 mg lozenge. If the first cigarette is smoked within 30 min of waking, start with the 4 mg lozenge. **Weeks 1–6:** 1 lozenge q 2 hr; **Weeks 7–9:** 1 lozenge q 2– 4 hr; **Weeks 10–12:** 1 lozenge q 4–8 hr.

## NEED TO KNOW

1. Do not use in nonsmokers, serious arrhythmias, angina, vasospastic disease, MI, active temporomandibular joint disease.
2. Use with caution in hypertension, peptic ulcer disease, oral or pharyngeal inflammation, gastritis, stomatitis, hyperthyroidism, insulin-dependent diabetes mellitus (type 1 diabetes), and pheochromocytoma.
3. Client must stop smoking completely when beginning to use the gum.
4. Have client chew gum slowly until it tingles; then, place it between the cheek and gum. When the tingle is gone, have client begin chewing again until the tingle returns. Repeat the process until most of the tingle is gone (about 30 min).
5. Advise client to place the lozenge in the mouth and allow it to dissolve slowly (20–30 min). Minimize swallowing. Client should not chew or swallow the lozenge. A warm or tingling sensation may be felt. Advise to occasionally move the lozenge from one side of the mouth to the other.
6. Advise client not to eat or drink for 15 min before chewing the nicotine gum or while using the lozenge.
7. Do not use more than 24 pieces/day. Stop using nicotine gum at the end of 12 weeks.
8. Acidic beverages, such as coffee, juices, soft drinks, and wine, interfere with buccal absorption of nicotine; thus, avoid eating and drinking 15 min before and during chewing.

# Nicotine transdermal system
(NIK-oh-teen)

**D**

**OTC:** Nicoderm CQ Step 1, Step 2, and Step 3., Nicotine Transdermal System Step 1, Step 2, and Step 3., Nicotrol Step 1, Step 2, and Step 3.

**CLASSIFICATION(S):** Smoking deterrent

**USES:** As an aid to stopping smoking for the relief of nicotine withdrawal symptoms. Should be used in conjunction with a comprehensive behavioral smoking cessation program.

**ACTION/KINETICS:** Nicotine transdermal system is a multilayered film that provides systemic delivery of varying amounts of nicotine over a 24-hr period after applying to the skin. Nicotine's reinforcing activity is due to stimulation of the cortex (via the locus ceruleus), producing increased alertness and cognitive performance and a 'reward' effect due to an action in the limbic system. **Time to peak levels:** 2–12 hr. **Peak plasma levels:** 5–17 ng/mL. **t½:** 3–4 hr. Metabolized in the liver to a large number of metabolites, all of which are less active than nicotine.

**SIDE EFFECTS:** Erythema, pruritus, or burning at site of application; headache. *NOTE:* The incidence of side effects is complicated by the fact that clients manifest effects of nicotine withdrawal or by concurrent smoking.

**DOSAGE: Transdermal System** NICODERM CQ, NICOTINE TRANSDERMAL SYSTEM

*Smoking deterrent.*

**Adults:** 21 mg/day for the first 6 weeks, 14 mg/day for the next 2 weeks, and 7 mg/day for the last 2 weeks. Total course of therapy: 8–10 weeks. Start with 14 mg/day for 6 weeks for those who smoke fewer than 10 cigarettes/day. Decrease dose to 7 mg/day for the final 2 weeks.

**DOSAGE: Transdermal System** NICOTROL

*Smoking deterrent.*

**Adults:** 15 mg/16 hr for the first 6 weeks, 10 mg/16 hr for the next 2 weeks, and 5 mg/16 hr for the last 2 weeks. Total course of therapy: 10 weeks.

## NEED TO KNOW

1. Do not use in those with heart disease, hypertension, a recent MI, severe or worsening angina pectoris, those taking certain antidepressants or antiasthmatic drugs, or in severe renal impairment.

2. Use with caution in clients with hyperthyroidism, pheochromocytoma, insulin-dependent diabetes mellitus (type 1 diabetes) (nicotine causes the release of catecholamines), in active peptic ulcers, in accelerated hypertension.

3. The goal of therapy with nicotine transdermal systems is complete abstinence. If still smoking by the fourth week of therapy, discontinue treatment.

4. Use extreme caution during application; remove old patch first then immediately apply the new one to a nonhairy, dry skin site. Avoid eye contact. These systems can be a skin irritant and cause contact dermatitis. Report any persistent skin irritations such as redness, swelling, or itching at the application site as well as any generalized skin reactions such as large red skin elevations, or a generalized rash; remove system.

5. Symptoms of nicotine withdrawal include craving, nervousness, restlessness, irritability, mood lability, anxiety, drowsiness, sleep disturbances, impaired concentration, increased appetite, headache, myalgia, constipation, fatigue, and weight gain; report as dosage may require adjustment.

6. Change site of application daily; do not reuse same site for 1 week. With Nicotrol, remove patch at bedtime and apply upon arising.

7. For Nicoderm CQ, remove the used system after 16–24 hr and apply a new system to alternate skin site. Do not leave the patch on for more than 24 hr as skin irritation may occur and potency is lost. Apply at the same time each day. If vivid

dreams or other sleep disturbances, patch may be removed at bedtime and a new patch applied in the morning.

8. For Nicotrol, apply a new system each day upon waking and remove at bedtime. If forget to remove patch at bedtime, vivid dreams or other sleep disturbances may result. Do not wear patch more than 16 hr.

9. If therapy is unsuccessful after 4 weeks, discontinue and identify reasons for failure so that a later attempt may be more successful.

## Nitroglycerin sublingual     C
(nye-troh-**GLIH**-sir-in)
**Rx:** NitroQuick, Nitrostat, NitroTab.

**CLASSIFICATION(S):** Vasodilator, coronary

**USES:** Acute relief or prophylaxis of angina pectoris caused by coronary artery disease.

**ACTION/KINETICS:** Relax vascular smooth muscle by stimulating production of intracellular cyclic guanosine monophosphate. Dilation of postcapillary vessels decreases venous return to the heart due to pooling of blood; thus, LV end-diastolic pressure (preload) is reduced. Relaxation of arterioles results in a decreased systemic vascular resistance and arterial pressure (afterload). Rapidly absorbed. **Onset:** 1–3 min; **mean peak plasma levels:** 6–7 min. **duration:** 30–60 min. **t ½, elimination:** About 2–3 min. Rapidly metabolized to dinitrates and mononitrates by a liver reductase enzyme. Also metabolized by red blood cells and vascular walls.

**SIDE EFFECTS:** Headache (may be severe and persistent), dizziness, palpitations, vertigo, weakness, postural hypotension, syncope.

## DOSAGE: Tablets, Sublingual

**Adults:** Dissolve 1 tablet under the tongue or in the buccal pouch at first sign of attack; may be repeated in 5 min if necessary (no more than 3 tablets should be taken within 15 min).

For prophylaxis, tablets may be taken 5–10 min prior to activities that may precipitate an attack.

**NEED TO KNOW**

1. Sit down and place sublingual tablet under the tongue and allow to dissolve; do not swallow until entirely dissolved. May sting when it comes in contact with the mucosa.
2. Take 5–10 min *before* stressful activity, i.e., exercise, sex. Check with provider, may consider additional dose before anticipated stressful activity or if chest pain at night.
3. Report immediately if pain is not controlled with prescribed dosage (usually 1 tab q 5 min × 3). Call 911 or for an ambulance as directed by provider if relief not attained.
4. Date sublingual container upon opening. Protect from moisture. Discard unused tablets if 6 months has elapsed since the original container opened.

---

## Omeprazole
(oh-**MEH**-prah-zohl)

**C**

**OTC:** Prilosec OTC. **Rx:** Prilosec.

**CLASSIFICATION(S):** Proton pump inhibitor
**USES: Rx.** (1) Short-term treatment of active duodenal ulcer. (2) With clarithromycin to treat duodenal ulcer associated with *H. pylori*. (3) Short-term (4–8 weeks) treatment of erosive esophagitis diagnosed by endoscopy. Maintain healing of erosive esophagitis. (4) Short-term (4–8 weeks) treatment of active benign gastric ulcer. (5) Long-term treatment of hypersecretory conditions (e.g., Zollinger-Ellison syndrome, multiple endocrine adenomas, systemic mastocytosis). (6) Treatment of heartburn and other symptoms associated with GERD. **OTC.** Frequent heartburn occurring 2 or more days/week. Not intended for immediate relief.
**ACTION/KINETICS:** Thought to be a gastric pump inhibitor in that it blocks the final step of acid production by inhibiting the $H^+/K^+$

ATPase system at the secretory surface of the gastric parietal cell. Both basal and stimulated acid secretions are inhibited. Serum gastrin levels are increased during the first 1 or 2 weeks of therapy and are maintained at such levels during the course of therapy. Absorption is rapid. **Peak plasma levels:** 0.5–3.5 hr. **Onset:** Within 1 hr. **t½:** 0.5–1 hr. **Duration:** Up to 72 hr (due to prolonged binding of the drug to the parietal $H^+/K^+$ ATPase enzyme). Metabolized in the liver and inactive metabolites are excreted through the urine. Consider dosage adjustment in Asians.

**SIDE EFFECTS:** Headache, abdominal pain, diarrhea, N&V, URTI, dizziness, rash. *AGRANULOCYTOSIS, ANAPHYLAXIS.*

---

## DOSAGE: Capsules, Delayed-Release (Rx)

*Active duodenal ulcer.*
> **Adults:** 20 mg/day for 4–8 weeks.

*Erosive esophagitis.*
> **Adults:** 20 mg/day for 4–8 weeks. Maintenance of healing erosive esophagitis, 20 mg/day. Controlled studies do not exceed 1 year.

*GERD without esophageal lesions.*
> **Adults:** 20 mg/day for up to 4 weeks.

*GERD with erosive esophagitis.*
> **Adults:** 20 mg/day for 4–8 weeks. In the occasional client not responding to 8 weeks of treatment, an additional 4 weeks of therapy may help. If there is a recurrence of erosive esophagitis or GERD, an additional 4–8 week course may be considered.

*Treatment of H. pylori .*
> **Adults:** The following regimens may be used: **Triple Therapy:** Omeprazole, 20 mg, plus clarithromycin, 500 mg, plus amoxicillin, 1,000 mg, each given twice daily for 10 days. If an ulcer is present at the beginning of therapy, continue omeprazole, 20 mg once daily, for an additional 18 days. **Dual Therapy:** Omeprazole, 40 mg once daily plus clarithromycin, 500 mg, 3 times per day for 14 days. If an ulcer is present at the begin-

ning of therapy, continue omeprazole, 20 mg daily, for an additional 14 days.

*Pathologic hypersecretory conditions.*
**Adults, initial:** 60 mg/day; then, dose individualized although doses up to 120 mg 3 times per day have been used. Daily doses greater than 80 mg should be divided. Continue treatment for as long as needed.

*Gastric ulcers.*
**Adults:** 40 mg once daily for 4–8 weeks.
**DOSAGE: Tablets, Delayed-Release (OTC)**

*Frequent heartburn, greater than 2 or more days/week.*
**Adults:** 20 mg tablet taken with a full glass of water once daily before the first meal of the day, every day, for 14 days. **Maximum daily dose:** 20 mg. Takes 1–4 days for the full effect. The 14-day course may be repeated q 4 months.

---

**NEED TO KNOW**

1. OTC use is contraindicated in those who have trouble with or pain swallowing food, are vomiting blood, or are excreting bloody or black stools.
2. Bioavailability may be increased in geriatric clients.
3. Symptomatic effects with omeprazole do not preclude gastric malignancy.
4. Take capsule at least 1 hr before eating and swallow whole; do not open, chew, or crush. Antacids can be administered with omeprazole.
5. For those who have difficulty swallowing capsules, add 1 tablespoon of applesauce to an empty bowl. Open omeprazole capsule and empty pellets onto applesauce. Mix pellets with the applesauce and swallow immediately. Do not heat or chew the applesauce and do not chew or crush the pellets. Do not store mixture for future use.
6. Report any changes in urinary elimination, pain, discomfort, or persistent diarrhea.

7. Avoid alcohol and OTC agents as well as foods known to cause GI upset/irritation.

## Ondansetron hydrochloride       **B**
(on-**DAN**-sih-tron)
**Rx:** Zofran, Zofran ODT.

**CLASSIFICATION(S):** Antiemetic

**USES: Oral:** (1) Prevent N&V resulting from initial and repeated courses of cancer chemotherapy, including cisplatin, greater than 50 mg/m$^2$. (2) Prevent N&V associated with initial and repeat courses of moderately emetogenic cancer chemotherapy. (3) Prevent N&V associated with radiotherapy in clients receiving either total body irradiation, single high-dose fraction to the abdomen, or daily fractions to the abdomen. (4) Prevent postoperative N&V. (5) Postoperatively in clients in whom N&V must be avoided, even when the incidence of postoperative N&V is low. **Parenteral:** (1) Prevent N&V associated with initial and repeat courses of emetogenic cancer chemotherapy, including high-dose cisplatin. Efficacy of the 32 mg single dose beyond 24 hr has not been determined. (2) Prevention of N&V postoperatively for those in whom nausea and/or vomiting must be avoided, even when the incidence of postoperative N&V is low.

**ACTION/KINETICS:** Cytotoxic chemotherapy is thought to release serotonin from enterochromaffin cells of the small intestine. The released serotonin may stimulate the vagal afferent nerves through the 5-HT$_3$ receptors, thus stimulating the vomiting reflex. Ondansetron, a 5-HT$_3$ antagonist, blocks this effect of serotonin. Whether the drug acts centrally and/or peripherally to antagonize the effect of serotonin is not known. **Time to peak plasma levels, after PO:** 1.7–2.1 hr. **t$\frac{1}{2}$, after IV use:** 3.5–4.7 hr; **after PO use:** 3.1–6.2 hr, depending on the age. A decrease in clearance and increase in half-life are observed in clients over 75 years of age, although no dosage adjustment is recommended. Significantly metabolized with 5% of a dose excreted unchanged in the urine.

**SIDE EFFECTS:** Diarrhea, headache, dizziness, malaise/fatigue, constipation, bradycardia, hypotension, drowsiness/sedation, anxiety/agitation, gynecological disorder, urinary retention, hypoxia, pruritus, pyrexia, shivers. *CLONIC-TONIC SEIZURES, ANAPHYLAXIS, BRONCHO-SPASM, SHOCK.*

## DOSAGE: IM; IV

*Prevent N&V due to chemotherapy.*

**Adults:** A single 32 mg dose or three 0.15 mg/kg doses. A single 32 mg dose is infused over 15 min beginning 20 min prior to the start of emetogenic chemotherapy. For the three-dose regimen, the first dose is infused over 15 min starting 30 min before the start of chemotherapy; the second and third doses are given 4 hr and 8 hr, respectively, after the first dose.

*Prevent postoperative N&V.*

**Adults:** 4 mg IV undiluted over 2–5 min immediately before induction of anesthesia or postoperatively as needed. Alternatively, 4 mg undiluted may be given IM as a single injection.

## DOSAGE: Oral Solution; Tablets; Tablets, Oral Disintegrating

*Prevent N&V associated with moderately emetogenic cancer chemotherapy.*

**Adults:** One 8 mg tablet or orally disintegrating tablet or 10 mL (equivalent to 8 mg ondansetron) oral solution twice a day. Give the first dose 30 min before treatment followed by a second 8 mg dose 8 hr after the first dose; **then,** 8 mg twice a day for 1–2 days after chemotherapy.

*Prevent N&V associated with highly emetogenic cancer chemotherapy.*

**Adults:** 24 mg once a day given 30 min before the start of single-day highly emetogenic chemotherapy, including cisplatin greater than or equal to 50 mg/m².

*Prevent N&V associated with radiotherapy.*

**Adults:** One 8 mg tablet or orally disintegrating tablet or 10 mL (equivalent to 8 mg ondansetron) oral solution 3 times per day. For total body irradiation give the above dose 1–2 hr before each fraction of radiotherapy administered each day.

*Prevent N&V in single high-dose fraction radiotherapy to the abdomen.*

**Adults:** One 8 mg tablet or orally disintegrating tablet of 10 mL (equivalent to 8 mg ondansetron) oral solution 1–2 hr before radiotherapy, with subsequent doses 8 hr after the first dose for each day radiotherapy is given.

*Prevent postoperative N&V.*

**Adults:** 16 mg given as a single dose of two 8 mg tablets or orally disintegrating tablets or 20 mL (equivalent to 16 mg ondansetron) 1 hr before induction of anesthesia.

**NEED TO KNOW**

1. With impaired hepatic function, do not exceed 8 mg PO or 8 mg IV daily infused over 15 min, 30 min prior to starting chemotherapy.
2. When used to prevent chemotherapy-induced N&V, dilute the 2 mg/mL injection in 50 mL of D5W or 0.9% NaCl injection and infuse over 15 min. The 32 mg premixed injection in 50 mL D5W requires no dilution.
3. Drug to be given exactly as prescribed q 8 h around the clock in order to ensure desired results. May be continued 1–2 days following radiation/chemotherapy to ensure prevention of N&V.
4. May cause drowsiness or dizziness. Do not perform activities that require mental alertness until drug effects realized.
5. Report any rash, diarrhea, constipation, altered respirations (bronchospasms), or loss of response.

# B

## Orlistat
(OR-lih-stat)

**OTC:** Alli. **Rx:** Xenical.

**CLASSIFICATION(S):** Antiobesity drug

**USES: OTC:** Weight loss in overweight adults 18 years of age and older along with a reduced calorie, low-fat diet. **Rx:** (1) Management of obesity, including weight loss and weight maintenance when used with a reduced-calorie diet. (2) To reduce risk for weight regain after prior weight loss. Orlistat is indicated for obese clients with an initial body mass index of 30 kg/m$^2$ or more, or 27 kg/m$^2$ or more in the presence of risk factors such as hypertension, diabetes, dyslipidemia.

**ACTION/KINETICS:** Reversible inhibitor of lipases resulting in inhibition of absorption of dietary fats. Acts in the lumen of the stomach and small intestine to form a covalent bond with the active serine residue site of gastric and pancreatic lipases. Inactivated enzymes are not available to hydrolyze dietary fat, in the form of triglycerides, into absorbable free fatty acids and monoglycerides. At therapeutic doses, it inhibits dietary fat absorption by about 30%. Weight loss was seen within 2 weeks of starting therapy and continued for 6–12 months. Metabolism occurs mainly in the GI wall. Unabsorbed drug is excreted through the feces. Weight loss caused by orlistat delayed the onset of type 2 diabetes in obese clients with impaired glucose tolerance.

**SIDE EFFECTS:** Headache; oily spotting, flatus with discharge; fecal urgency, fatty/oily stool, oily evacuation, increased defecation, abdominal pain/discomfort, influenza, URTI, ANAPHYLAXIS.

**DOSAGE: OTC: Capsules**

*Management of obesity.*

**Adults:** 60 mg 3 times per day with each meal containing fat, not to exceed 3 capsules/day.

*Management of obesity.*

**Adults:** 120 mg (1 capsule) 3 times per day with each main meal containing fat; give during or up to 1 hr after the meal. Doses greater than 120 mg 3 times per day have not been shown to produce additional benefit. Safety and effectiveness beyond 2 yr have not been determined.

**NEED TO KNOW**

1. Do not use in chronic malabsorption syndrome or cholestasis.
2. Use with caution in those with a history of hyperoxaluria or calcium oxalate nephrolithiasis.
3. When the Rx form is used, the client should be on a nutritionally balanced, reduced-calorie diet that contains about 30% of calories from fat. Distribute over 3 main meals the daily intake of fat, carbohydrate, and protein.
4. To ensure adequate nutrition, clients on either the OTC or Rx product should take a multivitamin containing fat-soluble vitamins and beta-carotene.
5. Weight lost due to orlistat may be accompanied by improved metabolic control in diabetics; this might require a reduction in dose of oral hypoglycemic drugs or insulin.
6. May cause GI S&S, gas with discharge, fecal urgency/incontinence, oily or spotty discharge, abdominal pain/discomfort, diarrhea. Should subside with continued use; report any persistent side effects.

# Oseltamivir phosphate    C
(oh-sell-**TAM**-ih-vir)
**Rx:** Tamiflu.

**CLASSIFICATION(S):** Antiviral
**USES:** (1) Prophylaxis of influenza A and B. (2) Treatment of uncomplicated acute influenza in adults who have been symptomat-

ic for 2 days or less. *NOTE:* Oseltamivir is not a substitute for early vaccination on an annual basis as recommended by the CDC.

**ACTION/KINETICS:** Hydrolyzed by hepatic esterases to the active oseltamivir carboxylate. May act by inhibiting the flu virus neuraminidase with possible alteration of virus particle aggregation and release. Drug resistance to influenza A virus is possible. Readily absorbed from the GI tract and extensively converted to oseltamivir carboxylate. About 75% of an oral dose reaches the systemic circulation as the carboxylate. **t$^{1}$⁄$_{2}$, oseltamivir:** 1–3 hr; **t$^{1}$⁄$_{2}$, oseltamivir carboxylate:** 6–10 hr. Over 99% is eliminated in the urine as oseltamivir carboxylate.

**SIDE EFFECTS:** N&V, headache, diarrhea, dizziness, abdominal pain, bronchitis. *TOXIC EPIDERMAL NECROLYSIS, STEVENS-JOHNSON SYNDROME, ANAPHYLAXIS (RARE).*

## DOSAGE: Capsules; Oral Suspension

*Prophylaxis of influenza.*

**Adults:** 75 mg once daily for at least 10 days. The recommended daily dose for prophylaxis during a community outbreak of influenza is 75 mg. For clients with a $C_{CR}$ between 10 and 30 mL/min, reduce dose to 75 mg every other day or 30 mg of the oral suspension every day. Begin treatment within 2 days of exposure to flu. For adults, safety and efficacy have been shown for use for 6 weeks or less.

*Treatment of influenza.*

**Adults:** 75 mg twice a day for 5 days. For clients with a $C_{CR}$ between 10 and 30 mL/min, reduce dose to 75 mg once daily for 5 days.

## NEED TO KNOW

1. Efficacy has not been determined in clients who begin treatment after 40 hr of symptoms, for prophylactic use to prevent influenza, for repeated treatment courses, or for use in those with chronic cardiac or respiratory disease.

2. Has not been shown to prevent bacterial infections. Has not

infections. Efficacy has not been determined for treatment or prophylaxis in immunocompromised clients.
3. Use the reconstituted solution within 10 days of preparation.
4. Do not double up on doses. Take any missed dose as soon as remembered. If the missed dose is remembered within 2 hr of the next scheduled dose, take at the usual time and resume usual schedule.
5. Tolerability may be enhanced if taken with food. May aggravate diabetes control.
6. May cause dizziness or lightheadedness; alcohol, hot weather, exercise, or fever may increase effects. To prevent dizziness, sit up or stand slowly, especially in the morning. Sit or lie down at the first sign of these effects.
7. An increased risk of confusion and unusual behavioral changes has been noted.

## Pantoprazole sodium
(pan-**TOH**-prah-zohl)

**B**

**Rx:** Protonix.

**CLASSIFICATION(S):** Proton pump inhibitor
**USES: PO:** (1) Short-term treatment (up to 8 weeks) in the healing and symptomatic relief of erosive esophagitis associated with GERD. An additional 8 weeks therapy may be indicated for those who have not healed after the initial 8 weeks of therapy.
(2) Maintenance of healing of erosive esophagitis and reduction in relapse rates of day- and night-time heartburn symptoms in those with GERD. (3) Long-term treatment of pathological hypersecretory conditions, including Zollinger-Ellison syndrome. **IV:** (1) Short-term (7–10 days) treatment of GERD associated with a history of erosive esophagitis, as an alternative to PO therapy in those who are unable to continue taking the delayed-release tablets.
(2) Pathological hypersecretory conditions associated with Zollinger-Ellison syndrome or other neoplastic conditions.

**ACTION/KINETICS:** Proton pump inhibitor that suppresses the final step in gastric acid production by forming a covalent bond to two sites of the $H^+/K^+$-ATPase enzyme system at the secretory surface of the gastric parietal cell. Results in inhibition of both basal and stimulated gastric acid secretion regardless of the stimulus. Duration greater than 24 hr due to binding to ATPase. Gastrin levels increase. Absorption begins only after the tablet leaves the stomach although it occurs rapidly. Absorption is not affected by antacids, although food may delay absorption up to 2 hr or longer. **Duration:** Over 24 hr. Extensively metabolized in the liver by the CYP system. **t½:** About 1 hr. Excreted in both the urine (71%) and feces (18%).

**SIDE EFFECTS:** Headache, diarrhea, flatulence, abdominal pain.

---

## DOSAGE: Tablets, Delayed-Release

*Treatment of erosive esophagitis.*

**Adults:** 40 mg once daily for up to 8 weeks; an additional 8 weeks therapy may be considered for those who have not healed after 8 weeks of treatment.

*Maintenance of healing of erosive esophagitis.*

**Adults:** 40 mg once daily.

*Pathological hypersecretory conditions, including Zollinger-Ellison syndrome.*

**Adults, initial:** 40 mg twice a day. Adjust dose as needed as dosage varies with each individual; up to 240 mg/day may be given, if needed. Treatment in some has continued for more than 2 years.

## DOSAGE: IV only

*GERD associated with a history of erosive esophagitis.*

**Adults:** 40 mg once daily for 7–10 days. Safety and efficacy for more than 10 days have not been shown.

*Pathological secretory conditions.*

**Adults:** Individualize dose. 80 mg q 12 hr. Doses higher than

240 mg or given for more than 6 days have not been evaluated.

1. Safety and efficacy of IV use as initial treatment for GERD have not been established.

2. Use with caution in severe hepatic impairment as there may be modest drug accumulation when dosed once a day.

3. Give by IV infusion through a dedicated line using the filter provided. The filter must be used to remove precipitate that may form when the drug is reconstituted or mixed with IV solution.

4. If administration is through a Y-site, the in-line filter must be positioned below the Y-site that is closest to the client. Flush the IV line before and after the administration of pantoprazole with either D5W or lactated Ringer's injection.

5. Do not give pantoprazole injection through the same line with other IV solutions.

6. Midazolam is incompatible with Y-site administration. Pantoprazole may not be compatible with products containing zinc.

7. Take as directed at the same time each day. Do not split, crush, or chew the delayed-release tablets; swallow whole. If unable to swallow a 40 mg tablet, two 20 mg tablets may be taken.

8. May take with or without food in the stomach. Antacid consumption will not affect absorption.

9. Avoid alcohol, aspirin or NSAIDs, and foods that may cause GI irritation.

10. Report abdominal pains, evidence of bleeding (bright blood or black tarry stools), and any unusual side effects, worsening of S&S, or lack of response; keep follow up appointments.

11. Avoid long-term consumption of drug; may mask GI malignancies.

**Paroxetine hydrochloride, Paroxetine mesylate** **D**
(pah-**ROX**-eh-teen)
**Rx:** Paxil, Paxil CR, Pexeva.

**CLASSIFICATION(S):** Antidepressant, selective serotonin reuptake inhibitor
**USES: Hydrochloride. Immediate- and Controlled-Release:**
(1) Treatment of major depressive episodes as defined in the DSM-III (immediate-release) or DSM-IV (controlled-release). (2) Panic disorder with or without agoraphobia (as defined in DSM-IV). (3) Treatment of social anxiety disorder (social phobia) as defined in the DSM-IV. Use does not include Pexeva. **Immediate-Release:**
(1) Obsessive-compulsive disorders (as defined in DSM-IV).
(2) Generalized anxiety disorder (as defined in DSM-IV); up to 24 weeks for maintenance therapy. (3) Posttraumatic stress disorder (as defined in DSM-IV). **Mesylate, Immediate-Release:**
(1) Treatment of major depressive disorder. Periodically evaluate the long-term usefulness. (2) Treatment of obsessive compulsive disorder (as defined in DSM-III-R). (3) Panic disorder (as defined in DSM-IV).
**ACTION/KINETICS:** Antidepressant effect likely due to inhibition of CNS neuronal uptake of serotonin and to a lesser extent norepinephrine and dopamine. Results in increased levels of serotonin in synapses. Completely absorbed from the GI tract; bioavailability is 100%. **Time to peak plasma levels:** 5.2 hr for immediate-release and 6–10 hr for controlled-release. **Peak plasma levels:** 61.7 ng/mL for immediate-release and 30 ng/mL for controlled-release. **t½:** 21 hr for immediate-release and 15–20 hr for controlled-release. **Time to reach steady state:** About 10 days for immediate-release and 14 days for controlled-release. Extensively metabolized in the liver to inactive metabolites. Approximately two-thirds of the drug is excreted through the urine and one-third is excreted in the feces.
**SIDE EFFECTS:** Insomnia, somnolence, nausea, dry mouth, asthe-

nia, headache, dizziness, tremor, excessive sweating, diarrhea/loose stools, constipation, abnormal ejaculation. *SEIZURES, POSSIBILITY OF SUICIDE ATTEMPT.*

## DOSAGE: Oral Suspension; Tablets, Immediate-Release

*Major depressive disorder.*

**Adults, initial:** 20 mg/day, usually given as a single dose in the morning. Some clients not responding to the 20 mg dose may benefit from increasing the dose in 10 mg/day increments, up to a maximum of 50 mg/day. Make dose changes at intervals of at least 1 week. **Maintenance:** Doses average about 30 mg/day.

*Panic disorders.*

**Adults, initial:** 10 mg/day usually given in the morning; may be increased by 10 mg increments each week until a dose of 40 mg/day (range is 10–60 mg/day) is reached. Maximum daily dose: 60 mg.

*Obsessive-compulsive disorders.*

**Adults, initial:** 20 mg/day; **then,** increase by 10 mg increments a day in intervals of at least 1 week until a dose of 40 mg/kg (range is 20–60 mg/day) is reached. Maximum daily dose: 60 mg.

*Social anxiety disorder.*

**Adults, initial:** 20 mg/day, given as a single dose with or without food, usually in the morning. Dose range is 20–60 mg/day.

*Generalized anxiety disorder.*

**Adults, initial:** 20 mg/day, given as a single dose with or without food, usually in the morning. Dose range is 20–50 mg/day. Change doses in 10 mg/day increments at intervals of 1 week or more. Doses greater than 20 mg/day do not provide additional benefit. **Maintenance:** Adjust dose to maintain the client on the lowest effective dosage; periodically reassess to determine need for continued treatment. Found to be effective for up to 24 weeks.

*Posttraumatic stress disorder.*

**Adults, initial:** 20 mg/day given as a single daily dose with or without food. Usual range: 20–50 mg/day. If needed, can increase dose by 10 mg/day at intervals of 1 week. **Maintenance:** Adjust dose to maintain the client on the lowest effective dosage; periodically reassess to determine need for continued treatment.

## DOSAGE: Tablets, Controlled-Release

*Major depressive disorder.*

**Adults, initial:** 25 mg/day given as a single dose with or without food, usually in the morning. Range: 25–62.5 mg/day. Change doses in increments of 12.5 mg/day, if needed, at intervals of at least 1 week. **Maintenance:** Average of 37.5 mg/day.

*Panic disorder.*

**Adults, initial:** 12.5 mg/day given as a single dose with or without food usually in the morning. If needed, increase dose by 12.5 mg/day at 1 week intervals, not to exceed 75 mg/day.

*Social anxiety disorder.*

**Adults, initial:** 12.5 mg/day given as a single dose, with or without food, usually in the morning. Usual range is 12.5–37.5 mg/day. If needed, increase dose at intervals of at least 1 week in increments of 12.5 mg/day, up to a maximum of 37.5 mg/day. **Maintenance:** Adjust dose to maintain the client on the lowest effective dosage; periodically reassess to determine need for continued treatment.

## NEED TO KNOW

1. Use with caution and initially at reduced dosage in elderly clients as well as in those with impaired hepatic or renal function, with a history of mania, with a history of seizures, in clients with diseases or conditions that could affect metabolism or hemodynamic responses.
2. Allow at least 14 days between discontinuing a monoamine

3. Even though beneficial effects may be seen in 1–4 weeks, continue therapy as prescribed. Effectiveness is maintained for up to 1 year with daily doses averaging 30 mg of immediate-release or 37.5 mg of controlled-release.
4. If discontinuing therapy, decrease dose incrementally. Abrupt cessation may cause dizziness, sensory disturbances, agitation, anxiety, nausea, and sweating.
5. Shake suspension well before using. May be given with or without food. Swallow controlled-release tablet whole; do not crush or chew.
6. Report excessive weight loss/gain and adjust diet and exercise to compensate.
7. Report any thoughts of suicide or increased suicide ideations. Advise family not to leave severely depressed individuals alone; possibility of a suicide attempt is inherent in depression and may persist until significant remission is observed.
8. Avoid prolonged sun exposure and use protection when exposed.

## Pioglitazone hydrochloride ■ C
(**pie**-oh-**GLIT**-ah-zohn)

**Rx:** Actos.

**CLASSIFICATION(S):** Antidiabetic, oral; thiazolidinedione
**USES:** (1) Type 2 diabetes as monotherapy as an adjunct to diet and exercise. (2) Type 2 diabetes in combination with a sulfonylurea, metformin, or insulin as an adjunct to diet and exercise. Used when diet and exercise plus the single drug does not adequately control blood glucose.
**ACTION/KINETICS:** Decreases insulin resistance in the periphery and liver resulting in increased insulin-dependent glucose disposal and decreased hepatic glucose output. Is an agonist for peroxisome proliferator-activated receptor (PPAR) gamma, which is

found in adipose tissue, skeletal muscle, and liver. Activation of these receptors modulates the transcription of a number of insulin responsive genes that control glucose and lipid metabolism. Reduces fasting plasma glucose 39–65 mg/dL from placebo and HbA1c 1–1.6% from placebo. After PO, steady state serum levels are reached within 7 days. **Peak levels:** 2 hr; food slightly delays the time to peak serum levels to 3–4 hr, but does not change the extent of absorption. Metabolized by CYP2C8, CYP3A4, and CYP1A1 to both active and inactive metabolites. Unchanged drug and metabolites are excreted in the urine (15–30%) and feces. **t½:** 3–7 hr (pioglitazone); 16–24 hr (total pioglitazone).

**SIDE EFFECTS:** URTI, headache, sinusitis, hypoglycemia, aggravated diabetes mellitus, tooth disorder, pharyngitis, myalgia, edema.

---

## DOSAGE: Tablets

*Type 2 diabetes as monotherapy.*

 **Adults:** 15 or 30 mg once daily in clients not adequately controlled with diet and exercise. Initial dose can be increased in increments up to 45 mg once daily for those who respond inadequately. Consider combination therapy for those not responding adequately to monotherapy.

*Type 2 diabetes as combination therapy.*

 **Adults: If combined with a sulfonylurea:** Initiate pioglitazone at 15 or 30 mg once daily. The current sulfonylurea dose can be continued unless hypoglycemia occurs; then, reduce the sulfonylurea dose. **If combined with metformin:** Initiate pioglitazone at 15 or 30 mg once daily. The current metformin dose can be continued; it is unlikely the metformin dose will have to be adjusted due to hypoglycemia. **If combined with insulin:** Initiate pioglitazone at 15 or 30 mg once daily. The current insulin dose can be continued unless hypoglycemia occurs or plasma glucose levels decrease to less than 100 mg/dL; then, decrease the insulin dose by 10 to 25%. Individualize further dosage adjustments based on glucose-lowering response. NOTE: Daily dose of pioglitazone should not exceed 45 mg.

**NEED TO KNOW**

1. Thiazolidinediones, including pioglitazone, cause or exacerbate CHF in some clients.
2. Do not use in clients with type 1 diabetes, diabetic ketoacidosis, active liver disease, with ALT levels that exceed 2.5 times upper limit of normal, in clients with NYHA Class III or IV heart failure.
3. Increased risk for hypoglycemia when combined with insulin or other oral hypoglycemics.
4. It is recommended that clients be treated with pioglitazone for a period of time (3 months) adequate to evaluate changes in HbA1c unless glycemic control deteriorates.
5. Take once daily without regard to meals. Follow dietary guidelines, perform regular exercise, weight loss, dietary restrictions and other lifestyle changes consistent with controlling diabetes.
6. May cause swelling of extremities, resumption of ovulation (in premenopausal, anovulatory women), and hypoglycemia. Report if dark urine, abdominal pain, fatigue, or unexplained N&V occur.
7. Immediately report onset of an unusually rapid increase in weight or extremity swelling, shortness of breath, or other symptoms of heart failure.

---

**Pramipexole**                                                    **C**
(prah-mih-**PEX**-ohl)
**Rx:** Mirapex.

CLASSIFICATION(S): Antiparkinson drug
USES: (1) Signs and symptoms of idiopathic Parkinson's disease.
(2) Moderate to severe restless leg syndrome.
ACTION/KINETICS: Thought to act by stimulating dopamine (es-

pecially D$_3$) receptors in striatum. Rapidly absorbed. **Peak levels:** 2 hr. Food increases time for maximum levels to occur. **t$^{1}\!/_{2}$, terminal:** About 8 hr (12 hr in geriatric clients). Excreted mainly unchanged in urine. Clearance decreases with age.

**SIDE EFFECTS:** Postural hypotension, dyskinesia, extrapyramidal syndrome, insomnia, dizziness, hallucinations, abnormal dreams, confusion, constipation, dry mouth, accidental injury, asthenia.

---

**DOSAGE: Tablets**

*Parkinsonism.*

**Adults: Week 1:** 0.125 mg 3 times per day. **Week 2:** 0.25 mg 3 times per day. **Week 3:** 0.5 mg 3 times per day. **Week 4:** 0.75 mg 3 times per day. **Week 5:** 1 mg 3 times per day. **Week 6:** 1.25 mg 3 times per day. **Week 7:** 1.5 mg 3 times per day. **Maintenance:** 1.5–4.5 mg/day in equally divided doses 3 times per day with or without concomitant levodopa (about 800 mg/day). **Impaired renal function: C$_{CR}$ greater than 60 mL/min:** Start with 0.125 mg 3 times per day, up to maximum of 1.5 mg 3 times per day. **C$_{CR}$ 35–59 mL/min:** Start with 0.125 mg twice/day, up to maximum of 1.5 mg twice/day. **C$_{CR}$ 15–34 mL/min:** Start with 0.125 mg once daily, up to maximum of 1.5 mg once daily. **C$_{CR}$ less than 15 mL/min and hemodialysis clients:** Pramipexole not adequately studied in this group.

*Restless legs syndrome.*

**Adults, initial:** 0.125 mg once daily 2–3 hr before bedtime. For those requiring additional relief, the dose may be increased as follows after the initial dose is given for 4–7 days: 0.25 mg for 4–7 days followed by 0.5 mg for 4–7 days. Increase the duration between titration steps to 14 days in those with severe and moderate impaired renal function (C$_{CR}$ from 20–60 mL/min).

---

**NEED TO KNOW**

1. Possible sudden, overwhelming urge to sleep.

2. Gradually titrate dosage, increase the dose to reach a maximum therapeutic effect, balanced against the main side effects of dyskinesia, hallucinations, somnolence, and dry mouth.
3. Consider a decrease in levodopa dose if taken with pramipexole.
4. Do not increase dosage more frequently than every 5–7 days.
5. Discontinue pramipexole over a 1 week period.
6. May take with food to decrease nausea.
7. Rise slowly from sitting or lying position to prevent drop in BP.
8. May cause dizziness, fainting, blackouts, hypotension, sudden urge to sleep, and sedative effects.
9. May cause hallucinations; report if evident.
10. Avoid alcohol and any other CNS depressants; may exaggerate drowsiness and dizziness.

---

## Pravastatin sodium    X
(prah-vah-**STAH**-tin)
**Rx:** Pravachol.

**CLASSIFICATION(S):** Antihyperlipidemic, HMG-CoA reductase inhibitor

**USES:** (1) Adjunct to diet for reducing elevated total and LDL cholesterol and triglyceride levels in clients with primary hypercholesterolemia (type IIa and IIb) and mixed dyslipidemia when the response to a diet with restricted saturated fat and cholesterol has not been effective. Treat elevated serum triglyceride levels (Fredrickson Type IV) and primary dysbetalipoproteinemia (Fredrickson Type III). Reduction of apolipoprotein B serum levels. (2) Reduce the risk of recurrent MI in those with previous MI and normal cholesterol levels; reduce risk of undergoing myocardial revascularization procedures; reduce risk of stroke or TIA. (3) Reduce risk of MI in hypercholesterolemia without evidence of coronary heart disease; reduce risk of CV mortality with no increase in death from noncardiovascular causes. (4) Slow the progression of coronary atherosclerosis and reduce risk of acute coronary events in hypercholesterolemia with clinically evident CAD, including prior MI.

**ACTION/KINETICS:** Competitively inhibits HMG-CoA reductase; this enzyme catalyzes the early rate-limiting step in the synthesis of cholesterol. Thus, cholesterol synthesis is inhibited/decreased. Decreases total cholesterol, triglycerides, LDL, and VLDL and increases HDL. Drug increases survival in heart transplant recipients. Rapidly absorbed from the GI tract; absolute bioavailability is 17%. **Peak plasma levels:** 1–1.5 hr. Significant first-pass extraction and metabolism in the liver, which is the site of action of the drug; thus, plasma levels may not correlate well with lipid-lowering effectiveness. $t\frac{1}{2}$, **elimination:** 77 hr (including metabolites). Metabolized in the liver; excreted in the urine (about 20%) and feces (70%). Potential accumulation of drug with renal or hepatic insufficiency.

**SIDE EFFECTS:** Localized pain, N&V, diarrhea, abdominal cramps/pain, constipation, flatulence, fatigue, flu syndrome, common cold, rhinitis, rash/pruritus, cardiac chest pain, dizziness, headache. *PERIVASCULAR HEMORRHAGE, FULMINANT HEPATIC NECROSIS, HEPATOMA, ANGIOEDEMA, HEMOLYTIC ANEMIA, TOXIC EPIDERMAL NECROLYSIS, STEVENS-JOHNSON SYNDROME.*

---

**DOSAGE: Tablets**

*Antihyperlipidemic.*

**Adults, initial:** 40 mg once daily (at any time of the day) with or without food. A dose of 80 mg/day can be used if the 40 mg dose does not achieve desired results. Use a starting dose of 10 mg/day at bedtime in renal/hepatic dysfunction, in those taking concomitant immunosuppressants, and in the elderly (maximum maintenance dose for these clients is 20 mg/day).

---

**NEED TO KNOW**

1. Use with caution in clients with a history of liver disease or renal insufficiency.

2. In clients taking immunosuppressants (e.g., cyclosporine), begin pravastatin therapy at 10 mg/day at bedtime and titrate to higher doses with caution. Usual maximum dose is 20 mg/day.
3. Place on a standard cholesterol-lowering diet for 3–6 months before beginning pravastatin and continue during therapy, unless more than 3 risk factors.
4. Drug may be taken without regard to meals.
5. The lipid-lowering effects are enhanced when combined with a bile-acid binding resin. When given with a bile-acid binding resin (e.g., cholestyramine, colestipol), give pravastatin either 1 hr or more before or 4 hr or more after the resin. Only use this combination if further changes in lipid levels are likely to outweigh the increased risk of the drug combination.
6. Report unexplained muscle pain, tenderness, or weakness, especially if accompanied by malaise or fever.
7. Report severe GI upset, unusual bruising/bleeding, vision changes, dark urine, or light colored stools.
8. Avoid prolonged or excessive exposure to direct or artificial sunlight.

## Propranolol hydrochloride   C
(proh-**PRAN**-oh-lohl)

**Rx:** Inderal, Inderal LA, InnoPran XL, Propranolol Intensol.

**CLASSIFICATION(S):** Beta-adrenergic blocking agent
**USES:** (1) Hypertension, alone or in combination with other antihypertensive agents. (2) Angina pectoris when caused by coronary atherosclerosis (except InnoPran XL). (3) Hypertrophic subaortic stenosis (especially to treat exercise or other stress-induced angina, palpitations, and syncope); except InnoPran XL. (4) MI (except extended-release forms). (5) Adjunctive treatment of pheochromocytoma after primary therapy with an alpha-adrenergic blocker (except extended-release forms). (6) Prophylaxis of migraine (except InnoPran XL). (7) Essential tremor (familial or hereditary); ex-

cept extended-release forms. (8) Cardiac arrhythmias, including supraventricular, ventricular, tachyarrhythmias of digitalis intoxication and resistant tachyarrhythmias due to excessive catecholamines during anesthesia (except extended-release forms).

**ACTION/KINETICS:** Combines reversibly with beta-adrenergic receptors to block the response to sympathetic nerve impulses, circulating catecholamines, or adrenergic drugs. Manifests both beta$_1$- and beta$_2$-adrenergic blocking activity. Is also an antiarrhythmic, type II. Bioavailability is 30% for immediate-release and 9–18% for the long-acting product. **Onset, PO:** 30 min; **IV:** immediate. **Maximum effect:** 1–1.5 hr. **Duration:** 3–5 hr. **t$\frac{1}{2}$:** 2–3 hr (8–11 hr for long-acting). **Therapeutic serum level, antiarrhythmic:** 0.05–0.1 mcg/mL. Completely metabolized by liver and excreted in urine. Although food increases bioavailability, absorption may be decreased.

**SIDE EFFECTS:** Insomnia, anxiety, impotence, nervousness, fatigue, dizziness, drowsiness, lightheadedness, diarrhea, vision problems.

---

**DOSAGE: Capsules, Extended-Release; Oral Solution; Oral Solution, Concentrated; Tablets**

*Hypertension.*

**Adults, initial:** 40 mg twice a day or 80 mg of extended-release once a day; **then,** increase dose to maintenance level of 120–240 mg/day given in two to three divided doses or 80–160 mg of extended-release medication once daily. Do not exceed 640 mg/day.

*Angina.*

**Adults, initial:** 80–320 mg 2–4 times per day; or, 80 mg of extended-release once daily. **Dose range:** 80–320 mg 2, 3, or 4 times per day or 80–160 mg extended release once daily (gradually increase initial dose at 3–7 day intervals until optimum response is obtained). Do not exceed 320 mg/day.

*Arrhythmias.*

**Adults:** 10–30 mg 3–4 times per day given after meals and at bedtime.

*Hypertrophic subaortic stenosis.*

**Adults:** 20–40 mg 3–4 times per day before meals and at bedtime or 80–160 mg of extended-release medication given once daily.

*MI prophylaxis.*

**Adults:** 180–240 mg/day given in three to four divided doses. Do not exceed 240 mg/day.

*Migraine.*

**Adults, initial:** 80 mg extended-release medication given once daily or in divided doses; **then,** increase dose gradually to maintenance of 160–240 mg once daily or in divided doses. If a satisfactory response has not been observed after 4–6 weeks, discontinue the drug and withdraw gradually.

*Essential tremor.*

**Adults, initial:** 40 mg twice a day; **then,** 120 mg/day up to a maximum of 320 mg/day.

**DOSAGE: IV**

*Life-threatening arrhythmias or those occurring under anesthesia.*

**Adults:** 1–3 mg not to exceed 1 mg/min; a second dose may be given after 2 min, with subsequent doses q 4 hr. Begin PO therapy as soon as possible.

**NEED TO KNOW**

1. Do not use in bronchial asthma, bronchospasms including severe COPD.
2. Do not administer for a minimum of 2 weeks after MAO drug use.
3. Reserve IV use for life-threatening arrhythmias or those occurring during anesthesia.
4. If signs of serious myocardial depression occur, slowly infuse isoproterenol (Isuprel) IV.

5. May cause drowsiness; assess drug response before performing activities that require mental alertness.
6. Do not smoke; smoking decreases serum levels and interferes with drug clearance.
7. May mask signs of low blood sugar, such as a rapid heartbeat; monitor finger stick carefully.
8. Do not stop abruptly; may precipitate hypertension, myocardial ischemia, or cardiac arrhythmias.
9. Avoid alcohol and any OTC agents containing alpha-adrenergic stimulants or sympathomimetics.
10. Report persistent side effects, e.g., skin rashes, abnormal bleeding, unusual crying, or feelings of depression.

## Psyllium hydrophilic muciloid
(**SILL**-ee-um hi-droh-**FILL**-ik)

**OTC:** Fiberall, Genfiber, Konsyl, Metamucil, Modane, Natural Psyllium Fiber, Perdiem, Reguloid, Serutan, Syllact.

**CLASSIFICATION(S):** Laxative, bulk-forming

**USES:** (1) Prophylaxis of constipation in clients who should not strain during defecation. (2) Short-term treatment of constipation; useful in geriatric clients with diminished colonic motor response. (3) To soften feces during fecal impaction.

**ACTION/KINETICS:** The powder forms a gelatinous mass with water, which adds bulk to the stools and stimulates peristalsis. Also has a demulcent effect on an inflamed intestinal mucosa. Products may also contain dextrose, sodium bicarbonate, monobasic potassium phosphate, citric acid, and benzyl benzoate. Laxative effects usually occur in 12–24 hr. The full effect may take 2–3 days. Dependence may occur.

**SIDE EFFECTS:** Diarrhea, N&V, perianal irritation, bloating, flatulence, cramps.

**DOSAGE: Granules; Powder**

**Dose depends on the product. General information on adult dosage follows.**

*Laxative.*

**Adults:** 1–2 teaspoons 1–3 times per day; spread on food or take with a 8 oz of water or other liquid.

**DOSAGE: Effervescent Powder**

*Laxative.*

**Adults:** One packet in water 1–3 times per day.

**DOSAGE: Wafers**

**Adults:** Two wafers followed by a glass of water 1–3 times per day.

---

**NEED TO KNOW**

1. Do not use in severe abdominal pain or intestinal obstruction.
2. Mix powder with 8 oz of liquid just prior to administering; otherwise the mixture may become thick and difficult to drink. Wash down with another glass of water/juice.
3. The powder may be noxious and irritating when removing from the packets or canister. Open in a well-ventilated area and avoid inhaling particulate matter.
4. Take exactly as directed. Report lack of response, severe stomach pain, N&V, or intolerable side effects.
5. May take 12–24 hrs for desired response or up to 3 days. If taken before meals may reduce appetite.
6. Ensure adequate fluid intake and consume other dietary sources of fiber such as bran, cereals with fiber listed, fresh fruits, and vegetables.

**DOSAGE: Granules: Powder:**
**Dose depends on the product. General information on adult dosage follows.**
Laxative
**Adults: 1-2 teaspoons 1-3 times per day; spread on food or take with a lot of water or other liquid.**

**CLASSIFICATION(S):** Proton pump inhibitor

**USES:** (1) Short-term (4–8 weeks) treatment in the healing and symptomatic relief of erosive or ulcerative gastroesophageal reflux disease (GERD). (2) Maintenance of healing and reduction in relapse rates of heartburn symptoms in clients with erosive or ulcerative GERD. (3) Short-term (up to 4 weeks) treatment in healing and symptomatic relief of duodenal ulcers. (4) Long-term treatment of pathological hypersecretory symptoms, including Zollinger-Ellison syndrome. (5) Daytime and nighttime heartburn and other symptoms of GERD.

**ACTION/KINETICS:** Suppresses gastric secretion by inhibiting gastric $H^+/K^+$ ATPase at the secretory surface of parietal cells; it is a gastric proton-pump inhibitor. Blocks the final step of gastric acid secretion. **Peak plasma levels:** 2–5 hr. **t½, plasma:** 1–2 hr. **Onset:** Less than 1 hr. **Duration:** Over 24 hr. Extensively metabolized in the liver by CYP3A4 and CYP2C19. Excreted mainly in the urine.

**SIDE EFFECTS:** Headache, GI upset, diarrhea, insomnia, nervousness, rash, itching. *RECTAL HEMORRHAGE, CONVULSIONS, TOXIC EPIDERMAL NECROLYSIS, STEVENS-JOHNSON SYNDROME.*

---

**DOSAGE: Tablets, Delayed-Release**

*Healing of erosive or ulcerative GERD.*
> **Adults:** 20 mg once daily for 4–8 weeks. An additional 8 weeks of therapy may be considered for those who have not healed.

*Maintenance of healing of erosive or ulcerative GERD.*
> **Adults:** 20 mg once daily.

*Healing of duodenal ulcers.*
> **Adults:** 20 mg once daily after the morning meal for up to 4 weeks. A few clients may require additional time to heal.

*Treatment of pathological hypersecretory conditions.*

**Adults, individualized, initial:** 60 mg once a day. Adjust dosage to individual client needs (doses up to 100 mg/day and 60 mg 2 times per day have been used). Continue as long as clinically needed.

*Heartburn and other symptoms related to GERD.*

**Adults:** 20 mg once daily for 4 weeks. If symptoms do not resolve after 4 weeks, an additional course of treatment may be considered.

**NEED TO KNOW**

1. Greater sensitivity in some geriatric clients is possible.
2. Symptomatic response to therapy does not preclude presence of gastric malignancy.
3. Use with caution in severe hepatic impairment.
4. No dosage adjustment is needed in elderly clients, those with renal disease, or in mild to moderate hepatic impairment.
5. Swallow tablets whole with or without food; do not crush, chew, or split tablets.
6. Report unusual bleeding, acid reflux, abdominal pain, severe light-headedness, diarrhea, rash, or lack of effectiveness.
7. Avoid alcohol, NSAIDs, and salicylates; may increase GI upset.

---

**Raloxifene hydrochloride**  X
(ral-**OX**-ih-feen)
**Rx:** Evista.

**CLASSIFICATION(S):** Estrogen receptor modulator
**USES:** Prevention and treatment of osteoporosis in postmenopausal women. Not effective in reducing hot flashes or flushes associated with estrogen deficiency.
**ACTION/KINETICS:** Selective estrogen receptor modulator that reduces bone resorption and decreases overall bone turnover. Considered an estrogen antagonist that acts by combining with estro-

gen receptors. Has not been associated with endometrial proliferation, breast enlargement, breast pain, increased risk of breast cancer, or increased risk of heart attack and other heart problems. Also decreases total and LDL cholesterol levels. Absorbed rapidly after PO; significant first-pass effect. **t½:** 32.5 hr (multiple doses). Excreted primarily in feces with small amounts excreted in urine.

**SIDE EFFECTS:** Hot flashes, weight gain, nausea, dyspepsia, arthralgia, myalgia, sinusitis, pharyngitis, infection, flu syndrome.

## DOSAGE: Tablets

*Prevention and treatment of osteoporosis in postmenopausal women.*

**Adults:** 60 mg once daily.

## NEED TO KNOW

1. Do not use in active or history of venous thromboembolic events (e.g., DVT, pulmonary embolism, retinal vein thrombosis).
2. Use with caution with highly protein-bound drugs, including clofibrate, diazepam, diazoxide, ibuprofen, indomethacin, and naproxen.
3. May be taken without regard for meals.
4. Take supplemental calcium and vitamin D if daily dietary intake is inadequate.
5. Avoid prolonged immobilization and movement restrictions as with travel due to increased risk of blood clots. Stop 3 days prior to and during prolonged immobilization as with surgery or prolonged bed rest.
6. Drug is not effective in reducing hot flashes or flushes associated with low estrogen; does not stimulate breast or uterus.
7. Report pain in calves or swelling in legs, fever, insomnia, acute migraines, emotional distress, unexplained uterine bleeding, breast abnormalities, sudden chest pain, shortness of breath, or coughing up blood, as well as any vision changes.

## Ranibizumab
(ran-ih-**BIZ**-oo-mab)

**Rx:** Lucentis.

**CLASSIFICATION(S):** Selective vascular endothelial growth factor antagonist

**USES:** Neovascular (wet) age-related macular degeneration.

**ACTION/KINETICS:** Binds to the receptor-binding site of active forms of vascular endothelial growth factor A (VEGF-A). VEGF-A causes neovascularization and leakage and is thought to contribute to the progression of the neovascular form of age-related macular degeneration. The binding of ranibizumab to VEGF-A prevents the interaction of VEGF-A with its receptors on the surface of endothelial cells, reducing endothelial cell proliferation, vascular leakage, and new blood vessel formation. Small amounts are absorbed systemically. **t½, vitreous elimination:** 9 days.

**SIDE EFFECTS:** Conjunctival hemorrhage, eye irritation/pain, foreign body sensation in eyes, intraocular inflammation, increased intraocular pressure, retinal hemorrhage, blurred/decreased visual acuity, vitreous detachment/floaters, headache, arthralgia, nasopharyngitis, URTI, hypertension.

---

**DOSAGE: Intravitreal injection only**

*Neovascular (wet) age-related macular degeneration.*

**Adults:** Administer 0.5 mg (0.05 mL) by intravitreal injection once a month. Although less effective, treatment may be reduced to 1 injection every 3 months after the first 4 injections, if monthly injections are not feasible.

---

**NEED TO KNOW**

1. Do not use in ocular or periocular infections.
2. Using aseptic technique, all (0.2 mL) of the ranibizumab vial contents are withdrawn through a 5-micron, 19-gauge filter needle attached to a 1 mL tuberculin syringe. Discard filter needle after withdrawal from the vial; do not use for intra-

vitreal injection. Replace filter needle with a sterile 30-gauge × ½-inch needle for the intravitreal injection. Expel the contents until plunger tip is aligned with the line that marks 0.05 mL on the syringe.

3. Carry out intravitreal injection under controlled aseptic conditions, including use of sterile gloves, sterile drape, and a sterile eyelid speculum. Give adequate anesthesia and a broad-spectrum microbicide prior to the injection.

4. May experience red eye, eye pain, small specks in vision, sensation of something in eye, and increased tears. Other side effects may include high blood pressure, nose and throat infection, and headache.

5. Macular degeneration is usually seen in white females over 55 years old that have a family history, are obese, smoke, consume a diet low in minerals such as zinc and vitamins A, C, and E, and have cardiovascular disease.

## Ranitidine hydrochloride **B**
(rah-**NIH**-tih-deen)

**OTC:** Zantac 150 Maximum Strength Acid Reducer, Zantac 75 Acid Reducer. **Rx:** Zantac, Zantac EFFERdose.

**CLASSIFICATION(S):** Histamine $H_2$ receptor blocking drug
**USES:** **Rx:** (1) Short-term (4–8 weeks) and maintenance treatment of duodenal ulcer. (2) Pathologic hypersecretory conditions such as Zollinger-Ellison syndrome and systemic mastocytosis. (3) Short-term treatment of active, benign gastric ulcers and maintenance treatment after healing of the acute ulcer. (4) Treatment of GERD. (5) Treatment of endoscopically diagnosed erosive esophagitis and for maintenance of healing of erosive esophagitis. **IV.** (1) IV in some hospitalized clients with pathological hypersecretory conditions or intractable duodenal ulcers, or as an alternative to PO doses for short-term use in those who are unable to take PO medication. (2) Prevent paclitaxel hypersensitivity; reduce the incidence of GI hemorrhage associated with stress-related ul-

cers. **OTC:** (1) Relief of heartburn associated with acid indigestion and sour stomach. (2) Prophylaxis of heartburn associated with acid indigestion and sour stomach due to certain foods and beverages.

**ACTION/KINETICS:** Competitively inhibits gastric acid secretion by blocking the effect of histamine on histamine $H_2$ receptors. Both daytime and nocturnal basal gastric acid secretion, as well as food- and pentagastrin-stimulated gastric acid are inhibited. Weak inhibitor of cytochrome P-450 (drug-metabolizing enzymes); thus, drug interactions involving inhibition of hepatic metabolism are not expected to occur. Bioavailability is 50% after PO administration and 90–100% after IM. Food increases the bioavailability. **Peak effect, PO:** 2–3 hr; **IM; IV:** 15 min. **t½:** 2.5–3 hr. **Duration, nocturnal:** 13 hr; **basal:** 4 hr. **Serum level to inhibit 50% stimulated gastric acid secretion:** 36–94 ng/mL. From 30% to 35% of a PO dose and from 68% to 79% of an IV dose excreted unchanged in urine.

**SIDE EFFECTS:** Headache, abdominal pain, constipation, diarrhea, N&V. *AGRANULOCYTOSIS, AUTOIMMUNE HEMOLYTIC OR APLASTIC ANEMIA, BRONCHOSPASM, ANAPHYLAXIS.*

---

**DOSAGE: Rx: Capsules; Syrup; Tablets; Tablets, Effervescent**

*Duodenal ulcer, short-term.*

   **Adults:** 150 mg twice a day or 300 mg after the evening meal or at bedtime. A dose of 100 mg twice daily is as effective as the 150 mg dose in inhibiting gastric acid secretion. **Maintenance:** 150 mg at bedtime.

*Pathologic hypersecretory conditions.*

   **Adults:** 150 mg twice a day (up to 6 grams/day has been used in severe cases).

*Benign gastric ulcer.*

   **Adults:** 150 mg twice a day for active ulcer. **Maintenance:** 150 mg at bedtime.

*Gastroesophageal reflux disease.*
    **Adults:** 150 mg twice a day.

*Erosive esophagitis.*
    **Adults:** 150 mg 4 times per day.

*Maintenance of healing of erosive esophagitis.*
    **Adults:** 150 mg twice a day. **Maintenance:** 150 mg twice a day.

## DOSAGE: IM; IV

*Treatment and maintenance for duodenal ulcer, hypersecretory conditions, gastroesophageal reflux.*

    **Adults, IM:** 50 mg q 6–8 hr. **Intermittent bolus:** 50 mg q 6–8 hr (dilute 50 mg in 0.9% NaCl or other compatible IV solution to a concentration no greater than 2.5 mg/mL [20 mL]). Inject at a rate no greater than 4 mL/min (5 minutes). **Intermittent IV infusion:** 50 mg q 6–8 hr. Dilute 50 mg in 5% dextrose injection or other compatible IV solution to a concentration no greater than 0.5 mg/mL (100 mL) and infuse at a rate no greater than 5–7 mL/min (15–20 min) or use 50 mL of 1 mg/mL premixed solution and infuse over 15–20 min. Do not exceed 400 mg/day. **Continous IV infusion:** Add the injection to 5% dextrose injection or other compatible IV solution. Give at a rate of 6.25 mg/hr (e.g., 150 mg ranitidine injection in 250 mL of 5% dextrose injection at 10.7 mL/hr).

*Zollinger-Ellison clients.*

    **Adults, continuous IV infusion:** Dilute ranitidine in 5% dextrose injection or other compatible IV soution to a concentration no greater than 2.5 mg/mL with an initial infusion rate of 1 mg/kg/hr. If after 4 hr the client shows a gastric acid output of greater than 10 mEq/hr or if symptoms appear, increase the dose by 0.5 mg/kg/hr increments and measure the acid output. Doses up to 2.5 mg/kg/hr may be necessary.

## DOSAGE: OTC: Tablets

*Treat heartburn.*

    **Adults: Treatment:** 75 mg or 150 mg with a glass of water.

**Maintenance:** Use up to 2 times per day (up to 2 tablets in 24 hr).

*Prevent heartburn.*

**Adults:** 75 mg or 150 mg with a glass of water 30–60 min before eating food or drinking beverages that cause heartburn.

## NEED TO KNOW

1. Use with caution in the elderly and in clients with decreased hepatic or renal function.
2. Give antacids concomitantly for gastric pain although they may interfere with ranitidine absorption.
3. About one-half of clients may heal completely within 2 weeks; thus, endoscopy may show no need for further treatment.
4. The premixed injection does not require dilution; give by slow IV drip over 15–20 min. Do not introduce additives into the solution. If used with a primary IV fluid system, discontinue primary solution during drug infusion.
5. Take as directed with or immediately following meals. Wait 1 hr before taking an antacid. For EFFERdose tablets and granules, dissolve each dose in 6–8 oz of water before drinking. A liquid (syrup) is available if pills cannot be swallowed. Those who have feeding tubes may use this preparation.
6. Dizziness or drowsiness may occur.
7. Avoid alcohol, aspirin-containing products, and beverages that contain caffeine (tea, cola, coffee); these increase stomach acid. Avoid things that may aggravate symptoms, i.e., alcohol, aspirin, NSAIDs, caffeine, chocolate, and black pepper. Avoid herbals such as garlic, ginseng, ginkgo, or vitamin E with ulcer.
8. Report any evidence of yellow discoloration of skin or eyes, or diarrhea. Maintain adequate hydration. Report any confusion/disorientation, unusual bruising or bleeding, black tarry stools, diarrhea, or rash immediately.
9. Symptoms of breast tenderness will usually disappear after

several weeks, report if persistent and evaluate need to stop drug.

## Rasagiline
(rah-**SA**-jih-leen) **C**
**Rx: Azilect.**

**CLASSIFICATION(S):** Antiparkinson drug

**USES:** Treat signs and symptoms of idiopathic Parkinson's disease as initial monotherapy and as adjunct therapy to levodopa.

**ACTION/KINETICS:** Rasagiline is a potent, irreversible monoamine oxidase (MAO) inhibitor of MAO type B. The precise mechanism in treating parkinsonism is not known but may include an increase in extracellular levels of dopamine in the striatum. Rapidly absorbed. **Peak plasma levels:** 1 hr. Food does not affect the time to reach $T_{max}$, although $T_{max}$ and AUC are decreased by about 60% and 20%, respectively when the drug is taken with a high-fat meal. Undergoes almost complete metabolism in the liver mainly by CYP1A2. Excreted in the urine (62%) and feces (7%).

**SIDE EFFECTS: When used as monotherapy:** Headache, dyspepsia, flu syndrome, depression, fall, arthralgia, gastroenteritis, rhinitis, fever. **When used as an adjunct to levodopa therapy:** Dyskinesia, accidental injury, weight loss, postural hypotension, N&V, anorexia, arthralgia, abdominal pain, constipation, dry mouth, rash, ecchymosis, somnolence, paresthesia. *GI HEMORRHAGE, HEMORRHAGIC GASTRITIS, INTESTINAL PERFORATION, LARGE INTESTINE PERFORATION, HEART FAILURE, MI, ARTERIAL THROMBOSIS, CEREBRAL HEMORRHAGE, VENTRICULAR FIBRILLATION.*

**DOSAGE: Tablets**

*Idiopathic Parkinson's disease.*

**Adults, monotherapy:** 1 mg once daily. **Adjunctive therapy, initial:** 0.5 mg once daily; if satisfactory response is not obtained, may increase the dose to 1 mg once daily.

## NEED TO KNOW

1. Do not use with tyramine-rich foods, beverages, or dietary supplements and amines (from OTC cough/cold medications) to prevent a possible hypertensive crisis.

2. Do not use with meperidine, methadone, propoxyphene, tramadol, dextromethorphan, St. John's wort, mirtazapine, cyclobenzaprine, sympathomimetic amines (including amphetamines, nasal and oral decongestants, cold products, and weight-reducing products), other MAOIs, cocaine, and local or general anesthetics.

3. When used wtih levodopa, consider a decrease in the levodopa dosage, depending on individual client response.

4. Plasma levels of rasagiline may double in those taking concomitant ciprofloxacin or other CYP1A2 inhibitors. Thus, in such clients, use rasagiline, 0.5 mg/day.

5. May cause dizziness, drowsiness, lightheadedness, or fainting; alcohol, hot weather, exercise, or fever may increase these effects. To prevent them, sit up or stand slowly, especially in the a.m. Sit or lie down at the first sign of any of these effects.

6. Rasagiline should be discontinued at least 14 days before elective surgery.

7. If advised to stop taking rasagiline, wait at least 14 days before beginning to take certain other medicines (eg, medicines for depression, anxiety, pain, cough, congestion, weight loss, Parkinson disease; muscle relaxants). Confirm when to take new medicines after having stopped taking rasagiline.

8. Rasagiline may increase the risk of developing skin cancer. Report any skin changes (eg, change in color or thickness).

# Risedronate sodium
(rih-**SEH**-droh-nayt)

**Rx: Actonel.**

**CLASSIFICATION(S):** Bone growth regulator, bisphosphonate

**USES:** (1) Treatment of Paget's disease in men and women who (a) have a serum alkaline phosphatase level at least two times the upper limit of normal, (b) are symptomatic, or (c) are at risk for future complications from the disease. (2) Prophylaxis and treatment of postmenopausal osteoporosis. The drug increases bone mineral density and reduces the incidence of vertebral fractures and a composite end point of nonvertebral osteoporosis-related fractures. (3) Prophylaxis and treatment of glucocorticoid-induced osteoporosis in men and women taking the daily dosage equivalent of 7.5 mg or more of prednisone for chronic diseases. Adequate amounts of calcium and vitamin D must be given as well. (4) To increase bone mass in men with osteoporosis.

**ACTION/KINETICS:** Binds to bone hydroxyapatite and inhibits osteoclast activity, thereby preventing bone resorption. Appears to reduce fracture risk and reverse the progression of osteoporosis. Does not inhibit bone mineralization. Rapidly absorbed; food decreases absorption. **t½, initial:** 1.5 hr; **terminal:** 220 hr. Excreted unchanged in the urine.

**SIDE EFFECTS:** Infection, hypertension, chest pain, dizziness, headache, rash, abdominal pain, constipation, diarrhea, nausea, arthralgia, pharyngitis, edema, pain.

## DOSAGE: Tablets

*Paget's disease.*

**Adults:** 30 mg once daily for 2 months. Retreatment may be considered following posttreatment observation for at least 2 months if relapse occurs or if treatment fails to normalize serum alkaline phosphatase. For retreatment, the dose and duration of therapy are the same as for initial treatment.

*Prevention and treatment of postmenopausal osteoporosis.*

**Adults:** 5 mg once daily or one 35 mg tablet taken once

weekly or 75 mg taken on 2 consecutive days for a total of 2 tablets per month.

*Prevention and treatment of glucocorticoid-induced osteoporosis.*
**Adults:** 5 mg once daily.

*Osteoporosis in men.*
**Adults:** 35 mg once per week.

## NEED TO KNOW

1. May cause upper GI disorders, including dysphagia, esophagitis, esophageal ulcer, or gastric ulcer. Use with caution in those with a history of upper GI disorders.
2. Before starting therapy, treat hypocalcemia, other disturbances of bone and mineral metabolism.
3. Dosage adjustment is not necessary in clients with a $C_{CR}$ 30 mL/min or greater.
4. Take dose sitting or standing with a full glass of water at least 30 min before the first food or drink of the day. To facilitate delivery to the stomach and minimize esophageal irritation, take in an upright position with 6 to 8 oz of water. Avoid lying down for 30 min after taking drug. Mark calendar to ensure weekly dosing not missed.
5. If dietary intake inadequate, consume supplemental calcium and vitamin D. Antacids and calcium may interfere with drug; take them at different times during the day with food.
6. May experience nausea, diarrhea, bone pain, headache, and rash.
7. Report any swallowing difficulty, GI bleeding, throat/abdominal pain, muscle spasms, or dark-colored urine.

**CLASSIFICATION(S):** Treatment of Alzheimer's disease

**USES: PO, Transdermal:** (1) Mild to moderate dementia of the Alzheimer's type. (2) Mild to moderate dementia associated with Parkinson's disease.

**ACTION/KINETICS:** Probably acts by enhancing cholinergic function by increasing levels of acetylcholine through reversible inhibition of its hydrolysis by acetylcholinesterase. There is no evidence that the drug alters the course of the underlying disease. After PO, is rapidly and completely absorbed. Absorption from the patch is greatest from the back, chest, or upper arm. Administration with food delays absorption by 90 min, lowers $C_{max}$ by about 30%, and increases AUC by about 30%. **Peak plasma levels, after PO:** 1 hr; **from the patch:** 8 hr. Is rapidly and extensively metabolized by cholinesterase-mediated hydrolysis. **t½, elimination:** About 1.5 hr. Excreted mainly in the urine.

**SIDE EFFECTS:** N&V, dizziness, headache, diarrhea, anorexia, weight loss, abdominal pain, insomnia, confusion, asthenia, dyspepsia, accidental trauma, fatigue, UTI, tremor. *CONVULSIONS, CARDIAC FAILURE, MI.*

---

**DOSAGE: Capsules; Oral Solution**

*Mild-to-moderate dementia due to Alzheimer's disease.*

**Adults, initial:** 1.5 mg twice a day to minimize GI side effects. If the dose is well tolerated after a minimum of 2 weeks, may increase dose to 3 mg twice a day. Attempt subsequent increases to 4.5 mg and 6 mg twice a day only after a minimum of 2 weeks at the previous dose. If side effects are intolerable, discontinue treatment for several doses and then restart at the same or next lower dose level. If treatment is interrupted for longer than several days, reinitiate treatment with the lowest daily dose and titrate as described above. **Maximum dose:** 6 mg twice a day.

*Dementia associated with Parkinson's disease.*

**Adults, initial:** 1.5 mg twice a day; **then,** the dose may be increased to 3 mg twice a day and further to 4.5 mg twice a day and 6 mg twice a day, based on tolerability. There should be a minimum of 4 weeks at each dose. **Dose range:** 1.5–6 mg twice a day.

## DOSAGE: Transdermal Patch

*Dementia due to Alzheimer's disease or Parkinsons' disease.*

**Adults, initial:** 4.6 mg/24 hr. After a minimum of 4 weeks and if well tolerated, the dose should be increased to 9.5 mg/24 hr (the recommended effective dose). **Maintenance:** Increase doses only after a minimum of 4 weeks at the previous dose and only if the previous dose has been well tolerated. The maximum recommended dose is 9.5 mg/24 hr; higher doses offer no significant additional benefit but there is a significant increase in side effects.

## NEED TO KNOW

1. Use with caution in clients with a history of asthma or obstructive pulmonary disease.
2. Drugs that increase cholinergic activity may have vagotonic effects on the heart, and may cause urinary obstruction or seizures.
3. If side effects develop during treatment, discontinue treatment for several doses; restart at the lowest daily dose (to prevent severe vomiting) and titrate back to the maintenance dose.
4. The capsules and oral solution may be interchanged at equal doses.
5. Take with food in divided doses in the morning and evening.
6. If using the oral solution, remove the oral dosing syringe provided and withdraw the correct amount of drug from the container. Each dose of rivastigmine may be swallowed directly from the syringe or first mixed with a small glass of water, cold fruit juice, or soda.

7. Apply the transdermal patch once a day to clean, dry, hairless, intact healthy skin in a location that will not be rubbed by tight clothing. Do not apply to a skin area where cream, lotion, or powder has been applied recently.
8. Change the site of the transdermal patch application daily to avoid potential irritation, although consecutive patches can be applied to the same anatomic site (i.e., another site on the upper back). Do not use the same site within 14 days.
9. Drug may cause a high incidence of GI effects and N&V; monitor weight and report if loss significant so therapy can be reassessed. Stop drug and report any evidence of seizures, urinary obstruction, dizziness, and low heart rate.

## Ropinirole hydrochloride
(roh-**PIN**-ih-roll)

**C**

**Rx:** Requip.

**CLASSIFICATION(S):** Antiparkinson drug
**USES:** (1) Signs and symptoms of idiopathic Parkinson's disease, both as initial therapy and adjunctive therapy with levodopa. (2) Moderate to severe restless legs syndrome.
**ACTION/KINETICS:** Mechanism is not known but believed to involve stimulation of postsynaptic $D_2$ dopamine receptors in caudate-putamen in brain. Causes decreases in both systolic and diastolic BP at doses above 0.25 mg. Rapidly absorbed. **Peak plasma levels:** 1–2 hr. Food reduces maximum concentration. **t½, elimination:** 6 hr. First pass effect; extensively metabolized in liver.
**SIDE EFFECTS:** Dyskinesia, dizziness, somnolence, headache, hallucinations, falls, N&V, abdominal pain, pneumonia, fatigue, viral infection, increased sweating, edema, confusion.

**DOSAGE: Tablets**
*Parkinson's disease.*
  **Adults: Week 1:** 0.25 mg 3 times per day. **Week 2:** 0.5 mg 3 times per day. **Week 3:** 0.75 mg 3 times per day. **Week 4:** 1

mg 3 times per day. After week 4, daily dose, if necessary, may be increased by 1.5 mg/day on weekly basis up to dose of 9 mg/day. This may be followed by increases of up to 3 mg/day weekly to total dose of 24 mg/day.

*Restless legs syndrome.*
**Adults: Days 1 and 2:** 0.25 mg. **Days 3–7:** 0.5 mg. **Week 2:** 1 mg. **Week 3:** 1.5 mg. **Week 4:** 2 mg. **Week 5:** 2.5 mg. **Week 6:** 3 mg. **Week 7:** 4 mg. *NOTE:* Dose is to be taken once daily 1–3 hr before bedtime.

**NEED TO KNOW**

1. If taken with L-dopa, decrease dose of L-dopa gradually, as tolerated.
2. When discontinued, do so gradually over 7-day period. Reduce frequency of administration to twice daily for 4 days. For remaining 3 days, reduce frequency to once daily prior to complete withdrawal.
3. May be taken with or without food.
4. Change positions slowly to prevent sudden drop in BP. May cause dizziness, use caution; report if persists.
5. Avoid alcohol during therapy.

---

**Rosiglitazone maleate**
(**roh**-sih-**GLIH**-tah-zohn)
**Rx:** Avandia.

**C**

**CLASSIFICATION(S):** Antidiabetic, oral; thiazolidinedione
**USES:** (1) Monotherapy as an adjunct to diet and exercise to improve glycemic control in clients with type 2 diabetes. (2) In combination with a sulfonylurea, insulin, or metformin in clients with type 2 diabetes when diet and exercise and either single agent does not achieve adequate control. In clients inadequately controlled with a maximum dose of a sulfonylurea or metformin, add rosiglitazone to the regimen, rather than substitute for the sulfo-

hylurea or metformin. (3) in combination with a sulfonylurea plus metformin when diet, exercise, and both agents do not result in adequate glycemic control.

**ACTION/KINETICS:** Improves blood glucose levels by improving insulin sensitivity in type 2 diabetes insulin resistance. Active only in the presence of insulin. A highly selective and potent agonist for the peroxisome proliferator-activated receptor (PPAR)-gamma, which is found in adipose tissue, skeletal muscle, and liver. Activation of these receptors regulates the transcription of insulin-responsive genes involved in the control of glucose production, transport, and use. Fasting blood glucose decreases from 31–64 mg/dL from placebo and HbA1c decreases from 0.8–1.5% from placebo. **Peak plasma levels:** 1 hr (over 99% bioavailable). Food decreases the rate of absorption but not the total amount absorbed. **$t^1/_2$, elimination:** 3–4 hr. Extensively metabolized in the liver by CYP2C8 and CYP2C9; excreted in the urine (64%) and feces (23%).

**SIDE EFFECTS:** Headache, edema, back pain, injury, URTI, hyperglycemia, fatigue, sinusitis, diarrhea, anemia. *CARDIAC FAILURE, MI, DEATH FROM CV CAUSES.*

---

**DOSAGE: Tablets**

*Type 2 diabetes, monotherapy.*

**Adults, initial:** 4 mg once daily or in divided doses twice a day. If the response is inadequate after 8–12 weeks, the dose can be increased to 8 mg as a single dose once daily or in divided doses twice a day. A dose of 4 mg twice a day resulted in the greatest decrease in fasting blood glucose and HbA1c.

*Type 2 diabetes, combination therapy with sulfonylurea, insulin, or metformin.*

**Adults, initial:** 4 mg once daily or in divided doses twice a day. If the response is inadequate after 12 weeks, the dose can be increased to 8 mg (maximum daily dose) as a single dose once daily or in divided doses twice a day.

**NEED TO KNOW**

1. Thiazolidinediones, including rosiglitazone, cause or exacerbate CHF in some clients.

2. Rosiglitazone is not recommended in clients with symptomatic heart failure.

3. Do not use in clients with type 1 diabetes or diabetic ketoacidosis; with metformin in renal impairment; in clients with active liver disease; if serum ALT levels are 2.5 times upper limit of normal; in clients with NYHA Class III and IV heart failure.

4. Treatment may result in resumption of ovulation in premenopausal anovulatory clients with insulin resistance.

5. Use with caution in clients with edema, at risk for heart failure, or hepatic impairment. There is an increased risk of MI and CV events, especially in long-term users of insulin and those taking nitrates.

6. Doses of rosiglitazone higher than 4 mg daily in combination with insulin are not recommended. It is recommended that the insulin dose be decreased 10–25% if the client reports hypoglycemia or if the FBS concentrations decrease to less than 100 mg/dL. Make further adjustments based on glucose-lowering response.

7. Take once or twice daily as prescribed with meals (may also be taken without regard to meals). If dose missed may be taken at next meal.

8. Report if dark urine, abdominal pain, fatigue, or unexplained N&V occur. Also report any fever, sore throat, unusual bleeding/bruising, rash, or hypoglycemic reactions.

9. Report any new onset visual changes, SOB, chest pain, significant weight gain, or swelling of extremities.

**CLASSIFICATION(S):** Antihyperlipidemic, HMG-CoA reductase inhibitor

**USES:** (1) As an adjunct to diet in heterozygous familial and non-familial hypercholesterolemia. (2) Adjunct to diet in mixed dyslipidemia (Fredrickson Type IIa and IIb). (3) Adjunct to diet in elevated serum triglyceride levels (Fredrickson type IV). (4) Reduce LDL-C, total-C, and Apo-B in homozygous familial hypercholesterolemia (as an adjunct to other lipid-lowering treatments).

**ACTION/KINETICS:** Competitively inhibits HMG-CoA reductase; this enzyme catalyzes the early rate-limiting step in the synthesis of cholesterol. Thus, cholesterol synthesis is inhibited/decreased. Reduces total cholesterol, LDL-C, ApoB, and non–HDL-C in clients with homozygous and heterozygous familial hypercholesterolemia, nonfamilial forms of hypercholesterolemia, and mixed dyslipidemia. Also, reduces triglycerides and increases HDL-C. **Peak plasma levels:** 3–5 hr. About 10% metabolized by CYP2C9 to N-desmethyl rosuvastatin which has some activity. Excreted primarily (90%) in the feces. **t½, elimination:** About 19 hr. Severe renal or hepatic insufficiency significantly increase plasma levels.

**SIDE EFFECTS:** Myalgia, constipation, asthenia, abdominal pain, N&V, headache, diarrhea, dyspepsia, back pain, flu syndrome, UTI.

---

**DOSAGE: Tablets**

*Heterozygous familial and nonfamilial hypercholesterolemia, mixed dyslipidemia (Fredrickson Type IIa and IIb).*

**Adults:** Individualize therapy. **Initial:** 10 mg once daily (use 5 mg once daily for those requiring less aggressive LDL-C reductions or who have predisposing factors for myopathy). For clients with marked hypercholesterolemia (LDL-C greater than 190 mg/dL) and aggressive lipid targets, consider a 20-mg starting dose. After initiation and/or upon titration, analyze lipid levels within 2 to 4 weeks; adjust dosage accordingly. Reserve the 40-mg dose for those who have not achieved goal LDL-C at 20 mg.

*Homozygous familial hypercholesterolemia.*
**Adults, initial:** 20 mg once daily. **Maximum recommended dose:** 40 mg daily. Use rosuvastatin as an adjunct to other lipid-lowering treatments (e.g., LDL apheresis) or if other treatments are not available. *NOTE:* For clients with severe renal impairment ($C_{CR}$ less than 30 mL/min/1.73 $m^2$ not on hemodialysis), use an initial dose of 5 mg once daily; dosage should not exceed 10 mg once daily in these clients.

## NEED TO KNOW

1. Do not use in clients with active liver disease or with unexplained persistent elevations of serum transaminases.
2. Use with caution in clients who consume substantial amounts of alcohol and/or have a history of liver disease. Use with caution in those 65 years and older, in hypothyroidism, and renal insufficiency (all predispose clients to myopathy).
3. Temporarily withhold rosuvastatin in clients with an acute, serious condition suggestive of myopathy or predisposing to the development of renal failure secondary to rhabdomyolysis (e.g., sepsis, hypotension, major surgery, trauma, uncontrolled seizures and severe metabolic, endocrine, and electrolyte disorders).
4. Due to the possibility of myopathy and rhabdomyolysis, reserve 40 mg dose for clients who have not achieved their goal for LDL cholesterol with the 20-mg regimen.
5. Before beginning rosuvastatin therapy, try to control hypercholesterolemia with appropriate diet and exercise, weight reduction in obese clients, and treatment of underlying medical problems. Continue cholesterol-lowering diet during drug treatment.
6. The effect of rosuvastatin on LDL-C and total cholesterol may be enhanced if used with a bile acid binding resin such as

gemfibrozil. If gemfibrozil is used with rosuvastatin, limit the dose of rosuvastatin to 10 mg once daily.

7. Take once daily with or without food as directed. Do not use antacid for 2 hr after consuming drug.

8. Report any S&S of infections, unexplained muscle pain, tenderness/weakness (especially if accompanied by fever or malaise), surgery, trauma, or metabolic disorders as drug should be stopped.

---

## Sertraline hydrochloride
**(SIR**-trah-leen)
**Rx:** Zoloft.

**C**

**CLASSIFICATION(S):** Antidepressant, selective serotonin reuptake inhibitor

**USES:** (1) Major depressive disorder as defined in the DSM-III. (2) Obsessive-compulsive disorders as defined in DSM-III-R. (3) Panic disorder, with or without agoraphobia, as defined in DSM-IV. (4) Long-term use for posttraumatic stress disorder in men and women as defined in the DSM-III-R. (5) Acute and chronic treatment of social anxiety disorder (social phobia) as defined in the DSM-IV.

**ACTION/KINETICS:** Antidepressant effect likely due to inhibition of CNS neuronal uptake of serotonin and to a less extent norepinephrine and dopamine. Results in increased levels of serotonin in synapses. Steady-state plasma levels are usually reached after 1 week of once-daily dosing but are increased to 2–3 weeks in older clients. May cause slight sedation. **Time to peak plasma levels:** 4.5–8.4 hr. **Peak plasma levels:** 20–55 ng/mL. **Time to reach steady state:** 7 days. **Terminal elimination t½:** 1–4 days (including active metabolite). Washout period is 7 days. Food decreases the time to reach peak plasma levels. Undergoes significant first-pass metabolism. Excreted through the urine (40–45%) and feces (40–45%). Metabolized to N-desmethylsertraline, which has minimal antidepressant activity.

**SIDE EFFECTS:** Nausea, diarrhea/loose stools, headache, insomnia, somnolence, rash, dry mouth, dizziness, anorexia, abnormal ejaculation. *SEIZURES, SUICIDAL IDEATION OR ATTEMPT.*

## DOSAGE: Solution, Oral Concentrate; Tablets
*Major depressive disorder.*
**Adults, initial:** 50 mg once daily either in the morning or evening. Clients not responding to a 50 mg dose may benefit from doses ranging from 50–200 mg/day (average: 70 mg/day).

*Obsessive-compulsive disorder.*
**Adults:** 50 mg once daily either in the morning or evening; up to 200 mg/day may be required in some.

*Panic disorder.*
**Adults, initial:** 25 mg/day for the first week; **then,** increase the dose to 50 mg once daily. Up to 200 mg/day have been used.

*Post-traumatic stress syndrome.*
**Adults, initial:** 25 mg once daily. After 1 week, increase dose to 50 mg once daily. **Dose range:** 50–200 mg/day.

*Social anxiety disorder.*
**Adults, initial:** 25 mg once daily. After 1 week, increase to 50 mg once daily. **Dose range:** 50–200 mg/day. *NOTE:* Lower the dose or space dose frequency in those with hepatic or renal impairment.

## NEED TO KNOW
1. Do not use with MAOIs due to increased risk of QT prolongation.
2. Use with caution in hepatic or renal dysfunction, and with seizure disorders.
3. Plasma clearance may be lower in elderly clients.
4. The possibility of a suicide attempt is possible in depression and may persist until significant remission occurs.

3. Due to the long elimination $t_{1/2}$, do not increase dosage at intervals of less than 1 week.
6. Beneficial effects may not be observed for 2–4 weeks after starting.
7. At least 14 days should elapse between discontinuing a MAOI and starting sertraline therapy. Also, allow at least 14 days after discontinuing sertraline and starting an MAOI.
8. When discontinuing sertraline, a gradual reduction in dose rather than abrupt cessation is recommended whenever possible.
9. May take with/without food and in the evening if sedation is noted.
10. Loss of appetite, persistent nausea, and diarrhea with excessive weight loss should be reported.
11. Avoid OTC agents, alcohol, and any other CNS depressants. If alcohol consumed wait and take dose in the a.m.

## Sibutramine hydrochloride monohydrate (sih-**BYOU**-trah-meen)    C
**Rx: Meridia, C-IV.**

**CLASSIFICATION(S):** Antiobesity drug
**USES:** Management of obesity, including weight loss and maintenance of weight loss. Recommended for obese clients with initial body mass index of 30 kg/m$^2$ or more or 27 kg/m$^2$ in presence of hypertension, diabetes, or dyslipidemia. Use in conjunction with reduced-calorie diet.
**ACTION/KINETICS:** Main effect is likely due to primary and secondary amine metabolites of sibutramine. Inhibits reuptake of norepinephrine (NE) and serotonin (5HT), resulting in enhanced NE and 5HT activity and reduced food intake. Significant improvement in serum uric acid. Rapidly absorbed from GI tract. Extensive first-pass metabolism in liver. **Peak plasma levels of active metabolites:** 3–4 hr. **t$_{1/2}$, sibutramine:** 1.1 hr; **t$_{1/2}$, active metabolites:** 14–16 hr. Excreted in urine and feces.

**SIDE EFFECTS:** Headache, dry mouth, insomnia, nervousness, anorexia, constipation, increased appetite, nausea, dyspepsia, arthralgia, rhinitis, pharyngitis, sinusitis, back pain, flu syndrome, asthenia.

## DOSAGE: Capsules

*Obesity.*

**Adults, initial:** 10 mg once daily (usually in morning) with or without food. Use the 5 mg dose for those who do not tolerate 10 mg. If there is inadequate weight loss, dose may be titrated after 4 weeks to a total of 15 mg once daily. Do not exceed 15 mg daily.

## NEED TO KNOW

1. Do not use in clients receiving MAOIs, who have anorexia nervosa, those taking centrally acting appetite suppressant drugs, those with history of coronary artery disease, CHF, arrhythmias, or stroke.
2. Do not use with serotonergic drugs, such as fluoxetine, fluvoxamine, paroxetine, sertraline, venlafaxine, sumatriptan, and dihydroergotamine; also, do not use with dextromethorphan, meperidine, pentazocine, fentanyl, lithium, or tryptophan.
3. Use with caution in geriatric clients.
4. Use with caution in narrow angle glaucoma, history of seizures, or with drugs that may raise BP (e.g., phenylpropanolamine, ephedrine, pseudoephedrine).
5. May take with or without food.
6. Reevaluate therapy if client has not lost at least 4 pounds in first 4 weeks of treatment.
7. Allow at least 2 weeks to elapse between discontinuation of a MAOI and initiation of sibutramine and between discontinuation of sibutramine and initiation of a MAOI.
8. Report any signs of allergic reaction including rash or hives.
9. Avoid alcohol and OTC agents and report all prescribed medications to prevent interactions.

**CLASSIFICATION(S):** Drug for erectile dysfunction; drug for pulmonary arterial hypertension

**USES:** (1) **Viagra:** Erectile dysfunction. Has no effect in the absence of sexual stimulation. (2) **Revatio:** Pulmonary arterial hypertension (World Health Organization Group 1) to improve ability to exercise.

**ACTION/KINETICS:** Nitric oxide activates the enzyme guanylate cyclase, which causes increased levels of guanosine monophosphate (cGMP) and subsequently smooth muscle relaxation in the corpus cavernosum allowing inflow of blood. Sildenafil enhances effect of nitric oxide by inhibiting phosphodiesterase type 5 which is responsible for degradation of cGMP in the corpus cavernosum. When sexual stimulation causes local release of nitric oxide, inhibition of phosphodiesterase type 5 by sildenafil causes increased levels of cGMP in the corpus cavernosum and thus smooth muscle relaxation and inflow of blood resulting in an erection. Drug has no effect in absence of sexual stimulation. Rapidly absorbed after PO use; about 40% is bioavailable. Absorption is decreased when taken with high-fat meal. Increased plasma levels will occur in clients older than 65 years (40% increase in AUC), hepatic impairment (e.g., cirrhosis, 80% increase), severe renal impairment ($C_{CR}$ under 30 mL/min, 100% increase), and concomitant use of potent cytochrome CYP 3A4 inhibitors; in these clients, start with a 25 mg dose. $T_{max}$: 0.5–2 hr. **Onset:** About 30 min. **Duration:** 4 or more hr. Metabolized in liver by CYP3A4 (major) and CYP2C9 (minor). Is converted to active metabolite (N-desmethyl sildenafil). $t^{1}\!/_{2}$, **sildenafil and metabolite:** 4 hr. Excreted mainly in feces (80%) with about 13% excreted in urine. Reduced clearance is seen in geriatric clients.

**SIDE EFFECTS:** Headache, flushing, dyspepsia, nasal congestion, UTI, abnormal vision, diarrhea, dizziness, rash. *MI, SUDDEN CARDIAC DEATH, VENTRICULAR ARRHYTHMIA, CVA, SUBARACHNOID AND INTRACEREBRAL HEM-*

*ORRHAGE, PULMONARY HEMORRHAGE, CARDIAC ARREST, HEART FAILURE, CARDIOMY-OPATHY.*

## DOSAGE: Tablets

*Treat erectile dysfunction.*

**Adults: Viagra:** For most clients, 50 mg no more than once daily, as needed, about 1 hr before sexual activity. Take anywhere from 0.5 hr to 4 hr before sexual activity. Depending on tolerance and effectiveness, dose may be increased to maximum of 100 mg or decreased to 25 mg. The maximum recommended dosing frequency is once daily.

*Pulmonary arterial hypertension.*

**Adults: Revatio:** 20 mg 3 times per day. Take doses about 4–6 hr apart with or without food. Doses higher than 20 mg 3 times per day are not recommended.

## NEED TO KNOW

1. Do not use with organic nitrates (potentiate hypotensive effects) in any form or with other treatments for erectile dysfunction.
2. Do not use in men for whom sexual activity is not advisable due to underlying cardiovascular status.
3. Use with caution in clients with anatomical deformation of penis, in those with predisposition to priapism (e.g., sickle cell anemia, multiple myeloma, leukemia), in bleeding disorders or active peptic ulceration, and in those with genetic disorders of retinal phosphodiesterases.
4. Drug is potentially hazardous in those with acute coronary ischemia but not on nitrates; have CHF, borderline low BP, or borderline low volume status; are on complicated antihypertensive therapy with several drugs; are taking erythromycin or cimetidine; or have impaired hepatic or renal function.
5. Consider starting dose of 25 mg in the following situations associated with higher plasma levels of sildenafil: Over 65 years of age, mild hepatic impairment (Child-Pugh score of 5 or 6),

severe renal impairment (C$_{CR}$ less than 30 mL/min), and concomitant use of cytochrome CYP3A4 inhibitors (including erythromycin, itraconazole, ketoconazole, and saquinavir).

6. Do not exceed a maximum single dose of 25 mg sildenafil in a 48 hr period with concomitant use of protease inhibitors (e.g., ritonavir) for HIV disease.
7. Do not take 50 or 100 mg of sildenafil within 4 hr of alpha-blocker administration. A 25 mg dose may be taken at any time.
8. Take only as directed on an empty stomach 1–3 hr prior to intercourse.
9. May experience headache, flushing, upset stomach, stuffy nose, dizziness (from drop in BP), drowsiness, or abnormal vision (especially blue/green color discrimination); report any unusual, persistent, or bothersome effects.
10. Do not use more than once a day. Erections lasting more than 4 hr or painful erections lasting more than 6 hr require immediate care; penile damage may result.

## Simvastatin
(**sim**-vah-**STAH**-tin)     X
**Rx:** Zocor.

**CLASSIFICATION(S):** Antihyperlipidemic, HMG-CoA reductase inhibitor

**USES:** (1) Adjunct to diet to reduce elevated total and LDL cholesterol, apoprotein B, and triglyceride levels in hypercholesterolemia and mixed dyslipidemia (Fredrickson types IIa and IIb) when the response to diet and other approaches has been inadequate. (2) To increase HDL cholesterol in primary hypercholesterolemia and mixed dyslipidemia (Fredrickson types IIa and IIb)s. (3) Treatment of isolated hypertriglyceridemia (Fredrickson type IV) and dysbetalipoproteinemia (Fredrickson type III). (4) In coronary heart disease and hypercholesterolemia to reduce risk of total mortality by reducing coronary death; to reduce the risk of nonfatal MI; to reduce the risk for undergoing myocardial revascularization procedures; to reduce the risk of stroke or TIAs. **ACTION/KINETICS:** Competitively inhibits HMG-CoA reductase; this enzyme catalyzes the early rate-limiting step in the synthesis of cholesterol. Thus, cholesterol synthesis is inhibited/decreased. Decreases cholesterol, triglycerides, VLDL, LDL; and increases HDL. Does not reduce basal plasma cortisol or testosterone levels or impair renal reserve. **Peak therapeutic response:** 4–6 weeks. Approximately 85% absorbed; significant first-pass effect with less than 5% of a PO dose reaching the general circulation. $t^1\!/_2$: 3 hr. Metabolites excreted in the feces (60%) and urine (13%). Increased levels seen in those with hepatic and severe renal insufficiency. **SIDE EFFECTS:** Headache, abdominal pain/cramps, constipation, URTI, flatulence, diarrhea, asthenia, N&V, dyspepsia, myalgia, rash/pruritus. *RHABDOMYOLYSIS, PANCREATITIS, FULMINANT HEPATIC NECROSIS, HEPATOMA, ANGIOEDEMA, ANAPHYLAXIS, HEMOLYTIC ANEMIA, TOXIC EPIDERMAL NECROLYSIS, ERYTHEMA MULTIFORME (INCLUDING STEVENS-JOHNSON SYNDROME).*

---

**DOSAGE:** Tablets

*Hyperlipidemia, coronary heart disease.*

**Adults, initially:** 20–40 mg once daily in the evening; **maintenance:** 5–80 mg/day as a single dose in the evening. Consider a starting dose of 5 mg/day for clients on immunosuppressants (e.g., cyclosporine), those with LDL less than 190 mg/dL, or in those with severe renal insufficiency. Consider a starting dose of 10 mg/day for clients with LDL greater than 190 mg/dL. Consider a starting dose of 40 mg as an alternative for those who require a reduction of more than 45% in their LDL cholesterol (most often those with CAD). For geriatric clients, the starting dose should be 5 mg/day with maximum LDL reductions seen with 20 mg or less daily. Do not exceed 10 mg/day if used in combination with fibrates or niacin.

*Homozygous familial hypercholesterolemia.*

**Adults:** 40 mg/day in the evening or 80 mg/day in 3 divided doses of 20 mg, 20 mg, and an evening dose of 40 mg. Use as an adjunct to other lipid-lowering treatments (e.g., LDL apheresis) or if such treatments are unavailable.

**NEED TO KNOW**

1. Use with caution in clients who have a history of liver disease/consume large quantities of alcohol or with drugs that affect steroid levels or activity.
2. If no more than two risk factors, place on a standard cholesterol-lowering diet for 3–6 months before starting simvastatin; continue diet during drug therapy.
3. May give without regard to meals.
4. In clients taking cyclosporine or danazol together with simvastatin, begin therapy with 5 mg/day of simvastatin; do not exceed 10 mg/day simvastatin.
5. In clients taking amiodarone or verapamil together with simvastatin, the dose of simvastatin should not exceed 20 mg/day.
6. In clients with severely impaired renal function, start at 5 mg/day simvastatin; monitor closely.
7. Simvastatin is effective alone or together with bile acid sequestrants. Avoid use of simvastatin with gemfibrozil, other fibrates, or lipid-lowering doses (1 gram/day or more) of niacin unless the benefit of further alteration in lipid levels is likely to outweigh the increased risk of the drug combination. However, if simvastatin is used together with fibrates or niacin, monitor carefully; do not exceed 10 mg/day of simvastatin.
8. A low-cholesterol diet must be followed during drug therapy. Consult dietitian for assistance in meal planning and food preparation. Do not take with grapefruit juice. May enjoy grapefruit juice at other times during the day.
9. Report any S&S of infections, unexplained muscle pain, tenderness/weakness (especially if accompanied by fever or malaise), surgery, trauma, or metabolic disorders. Report as scheduled for lab tests, eye exam, and follow up visits.

10. May experience sun sensitivity; take precautions to avoid sun or use sun protection.

## Sumatriptan succinate
(**soo**-mah-**TRIP**-tan)

**C**

**Rx:** Imitrex.

**CLASSIFICATION(S):** Antimigraine drug
**USES:** (1) Acute migraine attacks with or without aura. Photophobia, phonophobia, N&V associated with migraine attacks are also relieved. Intended to relieve migraine, but not to prevent or reduce the number of attacks experienced. (2) Acute treatment of cluster headaches (injection only).
**ACTION/KINETICS:** Selective agonist for a vascular 5-HT$_1$ receptor subtype (probably 5-HT$_{1D}$) located on cranial arteries, on the basilar artery, and the vasculature of the dura mater. Activates the 5-HT$_1$ receptor, causing vasoconstriction and therefore relief of migraine. Transient increases in BP may be observed. Bioavailablity ranges from 14–19% after PO, nasal, or rectal use and 96% after SC administration. **Time to onset after SC:** 10 min after a 6 mg SC dose; **time to onset after PO:** 30 min; **time to onset after intranasal:** 15 min. **Time to peak effect after SC:** 12 min; **time to peak effect after PO:** 2.5 hr; **time to peak effect after intranasal:** 1–1.5 hr. **t½ distribution, after SC:** 15 min; **terminal t½:** 2.5 hr. Approximately 22% of a SC dose is excreted in the urine as unchanged drug and 38% as metabolites. Rapidly absorbed after PO administration, although bioavailability is low due to incomplete absorption and a first-pass effect (bioavailability may be significantly increased in those with impaired liver function). **PO, elimination t½:** About 2.5 hr. About 60% of a PO dose is excreted through the urine and 40% in the feces.
**SIDE EFFECTS:** Paresthesia, warm/cold sensation, chest pain/tightness, vertigo, malaise/fatigue, neck/throat/jaw pain or pressure, N&V, headache, dizziness. *SERIOUS AND/OR LIFE-THREATENING AR-*

## DOSAGE: SC

*Migraine headaches.*

**Adults:** 6 mg. A second injection may be given if symptoms of migraine come back but no more than two injections (6 mg each) should be taken in a 24-hr period and at least 1 hr should elapse between doses.

## DOSAGE: Tablets

*Migraine headaches.*

**Adults:** A single dose of 25, 50, or 100 mg with fluids as soon as symptoms of migraine appear. Doses of 50 or 100 mg may provide a greater effect than 25 mg. A second dose may be taken if symptoms return but no sooner than 2 hr following the first dose. **Maximum recommended dose:** 100 mg, with no more than 200 mg taken in a 24-hr period.

## DOSAGE: Nasal Spray

*Migraine headaches.*

**Adults:** A single dose of 5, 10, or 20 mg given in one nostril. The 20 mg dose increases the risk of side effects, although it is more effective. The 10 mg dose may be given as a single 5 mg dose in each nostril. If the headache returns, repeat the dose once after 2 hr, not to exceed a total daily dose of 40 mg. The safety of treating an average of more than 4 headaches in a 30 day period has not been studied.

---

### NEED TO KNOW

1. Do not use SC in clients with ischemic heart disease, history of MI, documented silent ischemia, Prinzmetal's angina, or uncontrolled hypertension.
2. Do not use with egotamine-containing products or MAOI therapy (or within 2 weeks of discontinuing an MAOI).
3. Do not use in clients with hemiplegic or basilar migraine.
4. Use with caution in clients with impaired hepatic or renal function, and in clients with heart conditions.

185

Q-T

5. Consideration should be given to administering the first dose of sumatriptan in the provider's office due to the possibility (although rare) of coronary events related to undiagnosed CAD.

6. Drug is used to terminate headaches not to prevent them. Take with plenty of water.

7. For tablets, take a single dose with fluids as soon as symptoms appear; a second dose may be taken if symptoms return, but no sooner than 2 hr after the first dose. If there is no response to the first tablet, do not take a second tablet without consulting provider.

8. With nasal spray, use one spray in one nostril at onset of symptoms; may repeat in 2 hr if headache returns but not if pain persists after initial dose.

9. Report if chest, jaw, throat, and neck pain occur after injection; this should be medically evaluated before using more Imitrex. Severe chest pain or tightness, wheezing, palpitations, facial swelling, or rashes/hives should be immediately reported.

10. Symptoms of flushing, tingling, heat, and heaviness, as well as dizziness or drowsiness may occur and should be reported before taking more sumatriptan.

11. Use caution; may cause coronary artery vasospasm. If angina occurs following dosing, report so the presence of CAD or a predisposition to Prinzmetal variant angina may be assessed before additional therapy. Other S&S suggestive of decreased arterial flow, such as ischemic bowel syndrome or Raynaud syndrome following therapy, should also be evaluated for atherosclerosis by provider.

**CLASSIFICATION(S):** Drug for erectile dysfunction

**USES:** Treat erectile dysfunction.

**ACTION/KINETICS:** During sexual stimulation, nitric oxide is released from nerve endings and endothelial cells in the corpus cavernosum of the penis. Nitric oxide activates the enzyme guanylate cylase causing an increased synthesis of cyclic guanosine monophosphate (cGMP) in the smooth muscle cells of the corpus cavernosum. The cGMP in turn causes smooth muscle relaxation, allowing increased blood flow to the penis, resulting in erection. Tissue levels of cGMP are regulated by both the rate of synthesis and degradation via phosphodiesterases (PDEs). The most abundant PDE in the human corpus cavernosum is the cGMP-specific phosphodiesterase type 5 (PDE5). Thus, tadalafil, which is a selective inhibitor of PDE5, enhances erectile function by increasing the amount of cGMP. **Onset:** About 30 min. **Maximum plasma levels:** 0.5–6 hr. **Duration:** 36 hr. Rate and extent of absorption are not affected by food. Predominantly metabolized by CYP3A4. **$t_{1/2}$, terminal:** 17.5 hr. Excreted mainly as metabolites in the feces (61%) and urine (36%).

**SIDE EFFECTS:** Headache, dyspepsia, nasal congestion, back pain, flushing, limb pain, myalgia, hypotension. *ANGINA PECTORIS, MI.*

---

**DOSAGE: Tablets**

*Erectile dysfunction.*

**Adults, initial:** 10 mg taken prior to anticipated sexual activity. Dose may be increased to 20 mg or decreased to 5 mg based on individual efficacy and tolerability. The maximum recommended dosing frequency is once per day for most clients.

---

**NEED TO KNOW**

1. Do not use, either regularly or intermittently, in those taking

any form of nitrates (due to potential for severe hypotension) or in those taking alpha-adrenergic blockers (except 0.4 mg daily of tamsulosin).

2. Do not use in men for whom sexual activity is inadvisable due to their underlying CV status.

3. Do not use in those with MI within the last 90 days, unstable angina or angina occurring during sexual intercourse, those with NYHA Class II or greater heart failure in the last 6 months, uncontrolled arrhythmias, hypotension, uncontrolled hypertension, those with a stroke within the last 6 months, and hereditary degenerative retinal disorders (including retinitis pigmentosa).

4. Older clients or those with significant left ventricular outflow obstruction or severely impaired autonomic control of BP may be more sensitive to the drug.

5. Use with caution in conditions that might predispose clients to priapism (e.g., such as sickle cell anemia, multiple myeloma, or leukemia) or anatomical deformation of the penis (e.g., angulation, cavernosal fibrosis, Peyronie's disease).

6. May be taken without regard to food.

7. Although clients 65 years and older may be more sensitive to the drug, no dosage adjustment is necessary.

8. The maximum daily dose should not exceed 10 mg in clients with mild or moderate hepatic impairment.

9. The maximum daily dose should not exceed 5 mg in clients with severe renal insufficiency or end-stage renal disease.

10. At least 48 hr should elapse between the last dose of tadalafil and beginning nitrate therapy; administer nitrates under close medical observation with appropriate hemodynamic monitoring.

11. The dose should be limited to 10 mg no more than once every 72 hr in those taking potent inhibitors of CYP3A4 (i.e., itraconazole, ketoconazole, ritonavir).

12. May experience headache, flushing, stuffy nose, GI upset, back/limb pain or muscle pains, dizziness (from drop in BP)

drowsiness, or abnormal vision, report any unusual, persistent or bothersome effects. If chest pain experienced seek medical care.

---

**Tamoxifen citrate** ■ **D**
(tah-**MOX**-ih-fen)
**Rx:** Soltamox.

**CLASSIFICATION(S):** Antiestrogen

**USES:** (1) Adjuvant treatment of axillary node-negative or node-positive breast cancer in women following total or segmental mastectomy, axillary dissection, and breast irradiation. (2) Reduce risk of invasive breast cancer following breast surgery and radiation in women with ductal carcinoma in situ. (3) Advanced metastatic breast cancer in men. (4) To reduce the incidence of breast cancer in high-risk women, taking into account age, previous breast biopsies, age at first live birth, number of first-degree relatives with breast cancer, age at first menstrual period, and a history of lobular carcinoma in situ.

**ACTION/KINETICS:** Antiestrogen believed to compete with estrogen for estrogen-binding sites in target tissue (breast); also blocks uptake of estradiol. The rate and extent of absorption of the oral solution is bioequivalent to that of the tablets under fasting conditions. **Steady-state plasma levels (after 10 mg twice a day for 3 months):** 120 ng/mL for tamoxifen and 336 ng/mL for N-desmethyltamoxifen (active metabolite). **Steady-state levels, tamoxifen:** About 4 weeks; **for N-desmethyltamoxifen:** About 8 weeks. $t\frac{1}{2}$ **for metabolite:** about 14 days. Tamoxifen is metabolized by CYP3A4, CYP2C9, and CYP2D6; tamoxifen and metabolites are excreted mainly through the feces. Objective response may be delayed 4–10 weeks with bone metastases.

**SIDE EFFECTS:** Flushing/hot flashes, altered/irregular menses, amenorrhea, vaginal discharge/bleeding, skin changes, fluid retention, mood changes. *PULMONARY EMBOLISM, THROMBOEMBOLIC DISORDERS, HEPATIC NECROSIS, STEVENS-JOHNSON SYNDROME.*

**DOSAGE: Oral Solution; Tablets**

*Breast cancer.*
  **Adults:** 10–20 mg twice/day (morning and evening) or 20 mg daily. If using the oral solution, give 10 mL for a 20 mg dose. Doses of 10 mg 2–3 times per day for 2 years and 10 mg twice a day for 5 or more years have been used. There is no evidence that doses greater than 20 mg daily are more effective.

*Reduction in incidence of breast cancer in high-risk women.*
  **Adults:** 20 mg/day for 5 years. There are no data to support use beyond 5 years.

*Ductal carcinoma in situ.*
  **Adults:** 20 mg/day for 5 years.

*Mastalgia.*
  **Adults:** 10 mg/day for 10 months.

**NEED TO KNOW**

1. Serious and life-threatening events associated with tamoxifen in the risk-reduction setting (women at high risk for cancer and women with ductal carcinoma in situ) include uterine malignancies, stroke, and pulmonary embolism.
2. Do not use in coumarin anticoagulant therapy or in women with a history of deep vein thrombosis (DVT) or pulmonary embolus.
3. Use with caution in clients with leukopenia or thrombocytopenia.
4. If hypercalcemia occurs (may occur in breast cancer with bone metastases), take appropriate measures; if severe, discontinue tamoxifen.
5. Increased bone and lumbar pain or local disease flares should subside; take analgesics as needed.
6. Consume 2–3 L/day of fluids to minimize hypercalcemia. Exercise to reduce calcium levels, improve circulation, and prevent thrombophlebitis. Perform ROM exercises if bedridden.
7. May experience 'hot flashes'; stay in cool environment. Wear

7. protective clothing, sunscreens, and sunglasses to prevent photosensitivity reactions.
8. Report headaches or decreased visual acuity; may be irreversible. Have regular eye exams, especially if higher than usual dosage.
9. Although the risk of breast cancer is significantly lowered, there is also an increased risk of endometrial cancer, pulmonary embolism, and DVT. Report any redness or tenderness in extremity, increased SOB, chest pain, mental confusion, or sleepiness to ensure no stroke or blood clot. Avoid smoking.

## Tamsulosin hydrochloride
(tam-**SOO**-loh-sin)
**Rx:** Flomax.

**B**

**CLASSIFICATION(S):** Alpha-adrenergic blocking drug
**USES:** Signs and symptoms of benign prostatic hypertrophy (BPH). Rule out prostatic carcinoma before using tamsulosin.
**ACTION/KINETICS:** Blockade of alpha$_1$-receptors (probably alpha$_{1A}$) in the prostate results in relaxation of smooth muscles in the bladder neck and prostate; thus, urine flow rate is improved and there is a decrease in symptoms of BPH. Food interferes with the rate of absorption. **t½, elimination:** 5–7 hr. Extensively metabolized in liver; excreted through urine and feces.
**SIDE EFFECTS:** Headache, dizziness, pharyngitis/rhinitis, abnormal ejaculation, shoulder/neck/back/extremity pain, asthenia, diarrhea, chest pain.

---

**DOSAGE: Capsules**
*Benign prostatic hypertrophy.*
    **Adult males:** 0.4 mg once daily given about 30 min after same meal each day. If, after 2 to 4 weeks, clients have not responded, dose can be increased to 0.8 mg daily.

**NEED TO KNOW**

1. Do not use to treat hypertension with other alpha-adrenergic blocking agents or in women.
2. Use with caution with concurrent administration of warfarin.
3. If dose is discontinued or interrupted for several days after either the 0.4 or 0.8 mg dose, start therapy again with 0.4 mg dose.
4. Take as directed; do not chew, crush, or open capsule. May take 30 minutes after the same meal each day to decrease GI upset. Report any loss of effectiveness or increased nighttime voiding.
5. May cause dizziness, drowsiness, and syncope. Change positions slowly to prevent sudden drop in BP.
6. Do not stop suddenly after prolonged use.

---

**Temazepam**  **X**
(teh-**MAZ**-eh-pam)
**Rx:** Restoril, **C-IV.**

**CLASSIFICATION(S):** Sedative-hypnotic, benzodiazepine
**USES:** Insomnia in clients unable to fall asleep, with frequent awakenings during the night, and/or early morning awakenings.
**ACTION/KINETICS:** Believed to potentiate GABA neuronal inhibition. The hypnotic action involves GABA receptors located in the CNS. The drug decreases sleep latency, the number of awakenings, and the time spent in the awake stage. Disturbed nocturnal sleep may occur the first one or two nights following discontinuance of the drug. Prolonged administration is not recommended because physical dependence and tolerance may develop. **Peak blood levels:** 1.2–1.6 hr. **t ½:** 10–17 hr. **Steady-state plasma levels:** 382 ng/mL (2.5 hr after 30-mg dose). Accumulation of the drug is minimal following multiple dosage. Metabolized in the liver to inactive metabolites.

**SIDE EFFECTS:** Drowsiness, dizziness, lightheadedness, incoordination.

---

**DOSAGE: Capsules**

*Insomnia.*

**Adults, individualize: Usual:** 15–30 mg at bedtime (7.5 mg may be sufficient for some to improve sleep latency). **In elderly or debilitated clients, initial:** 7.5–15 mg until individual response is determined.

---

**NEED TO KNOW**

1. Use with caution in severely depressed clients.
2. Geriatric clients may be more sensitive to the effects of temazepam.
3. Take only as directed; do not increase dose. May take several days before effects evident.
4. May cause daytime drowsiness. Avoid activities that require mental alertness until drug effects realized.
5. Avoid alcohol and CNS depressants; may increase CNS depression. Avoid tobacco; decreases drug's effect.

---

**Terazosin**                                                         **C**
(ter-**AY**-zoh-sin)
**Rx:** Hytrin.

**CLASSIFICATION(S):** Antihypertensive, alpha$_1$-adrenergic blocking drug
**USES:** (1) Hypertension, alone or in combination with diuretics or beta-adrenergic blocking agents. (2) Symptoms of benign prostatic hyperplasia (BPH).
**ACTION/KINETICS:** Blocks postsynaptic alpha$_1$-adrenergic receptors, leading to a dilation of both arterioles and veins, and ultimately, a reduction in BP. Both standing and supine BPs are lowered with no reflex tachycardia. Also relaxes smooth muscle of the prostate and bladder neck. Usefulness in BPH is due to alpha$_1$-re-

ceptor blockade, which relaxes the smooth muscle of the prostate and bladder neck and relieves pressure on the urethra. **Onset:** 15 min. **Peak plasma levels:** 1–2 hr. **t½:** 9–12 hr. **Duration:** 24 hr. Excreted unchanged and as inactive metabolites in both the urine and feces.

**SIDE EFFECTS:** Asthenia, dizziness, headache, somnolence, flu symptoms, nasal congestion, pharyngitis/rhinitis. *ARRHYTHMIAS, BRONCHOSPASM.*

**DOSAGE: Capsules**

*Hypertension.*

    **Adults, individualized, initial:** 1 mg at bedtime (this dose is not to be exceeded); **then,** increase dose slowly to obtain desired response. **Range:** 1–5 mg/day; doses as high as 20 mg may be required in some clients. Doses greater than 20 mg daily do not provide further BP control.

*Benign prostatic hyperplasia.*

    **Adults, initial:** 1 mg/day; dose should be increased to 2 mg, 5 mg, and then 10 mg once daily to improve symptoms and/or urinary flow rates. Doses greater than 20 mg daily have not been studied.

**NEED TO KNOW**

1. Geriatric clients may be more sensitive to the hypotensive and hypothermic effects of terazosin.
2. The initial dosing regimen must be carefully observed to minimize severe hypotension.
3. To prevent dizziness or fainting due to a drop in BP, take the initial dose at bedtime; the daily dose can be given in the morning.
4. If terazosin must be discontinued for more than a few days, reinstitute the initial dosing regimen if restarted.
5. When treating BPH, a minimum of 4–6 weeks of 10 mg/day may be needed to determine if a beneficial effect has occurred.

6. Take initial dose at bedtime to minimize side effects. Do not stop abruptly or titration must restart.
7. May cause dizziness or drowsiness.
8. Avoid symptoms of dizziness (drop in BP) by rising slowly from a sitting or lying position and waiting until symptoms subside.
9. Do not take within 2 hr of meds used for erectile dysfunction.

---

## Tolterodine tartrate        C
(tohl-**TER**-oh-deen)
**Rx:** Detrol, Detrol LA.

**CLASSIFICATION(S):** Urinary tract drug
**USES:** Overactive bladder with symptoms of urinary frequency, urgency, or urge incontinence.
**ACTION/KINETICS:** Acts as a competitive muscarinic receptor antagonist in the bladder to cause increased bladder control. Metabolized by first pass effect in the liver to the active 5-hydroxy-methyl derivative, which has similar activity as tolterodine. Rapidly absorbed with peak serum levels within 1–2 hr. Food increases bioavailability. Excreted in the urine.
**SIDE EFFECTS: Immediate-Release:** Dry mouth, headache, constipation, vertigo/dizziness, abdominal pain, diarrhea, dyspepsia, fatigue. **Extended-Release:** Dry mouth, headache, constipation, abdominal pain, somnolence, dyspepsia, xerophthalmia.

---

**DOSAGE: Capsules, Extended-Release**
*Overactive bladder.*
    **Adults:** 4 mg once daily taken with liquids and swallowed whole. May lower dose to 2 mg daily based on response and tolerability. For those with significantly decreased hepatic or renal function or who are taking drugs that are inhibitors of CYP3A4, the recommended dose is 1 mg twice a day.

**DOSAGE: Tablets, Immediate-Release**

*Overactive bladder.*

**Adults, initial:** 2 mg twice a day. Dose may be lowered to 1 mg twice a day based on individual response and side effects. Adjust dose to 1 mg twice a day in those with significantly reduced hepatic function or who are currently taking drugs that are inhibitors of CYP3A4.

**NEED TO KNOW**

1. Do not use in urinary retention, gastric retention, uncontrolled narrow–angle glaucoma, lactation.
2. Use with caution in renal impairment, in bladder outflow obstruction, in GI obstructive disorders (e.g., pyloric stenosis), and in those being treated for narrow–angle glaucoma.
3. Take as directed with or without food. Avoid alcohol and OTC antihistamines.
4. May experience dizziness/drowsiness, headache, blurred vision, dry mouth, and light sensitivity; use caution and report if persistent. If eye pain, rapid heart rate, SOB, urinary retention, rash, or hives appears notify provider.
5. Dry mouth symptoms may be relieved with sugar free candy/gum, ice/water, or saliva substitute.

---

## Triazolam       X
(try-**AYZ**-oh-lam)
**Rx:** Halcion, **C-IV.**

**CLASSIFICATION(S):** Sedative-hypnotic, benzodiazepine
**USES:** (1) Insomnia (short-term management, not to exceed 1 month). (2) May be beneficial in preventing or treating transient insomnia from a sudden change in sleep schedule.
**ACTION/KINETICS:** Decreases sleep latency, increases the duration of sleep, and decreases the number of awakenings. **Time to**

**peak plasma levels:** 0.5–2 hr. **t½:** 1.5–5.5 hr. Metabolized in liver; inactive metabolites excreted in the urine.
**SIDE EFFECTS:** Drowsiness, headache, dizziness, nervousness, lightheadedness, coordination disorders/ataxia, N&V.

---

**DOSAGE: Tablets**

*Insomnia.*

**Adults, initial:** 0.25–0.5 mg before bedtime. **Geriatric or debilitated clients, initial:** 0.125 mg; **then,** depending on response, 0.125–0.25 mg before bedtime.

**NEED TO KNOW**

1. Do not use concomitantly with itraconazole, ketoconazole, or nefazodone.
2. Geriatric clients may be more sensitive to the effects of triazolam.
3. Use caution when driving or operating machinery until daytime sedative effects evaluated.
4. Drug is for short-term use only; may cause physical and psychological dependence.
5. Avoid alcohol and CNS depressants. Report unusual side effects including hallucinations, nightmares, depression, or periods of confusion.

---

**Trimethoprim and Sulfamethoxazole**     **C**
(try-**METH**-oh-prim, sul-fah-meh-**THOX**-ah-zohl)
**Rx:** Bactrim, Bactrim DS, Bactrim IV, Cotrim, Cotrim D.S., Septra, Septra DS, Sulfatrim.

**CLASSIFICATION(S):** Antibiotic, combination
**USES: PO, Parenteral:** (1) UTIs due to *Escherichia coli, Klebsiella, Enterobacter, Pseudomonas mirabilis* and *vulgaris,* and *Morganella morganii.* (2) Enteritis due to *Shigella flexneri* or *S. sonnei.*
*(3) Pneumocystis carinii* pneumonitis in adults. **PO:** (1) Traveler's di-

arrhea in adults due to *E. coli.* (2) Prophylaxis of *P. carinii* pneumonia in immunocompromised clients (including those with AIDS). (3) Acute exacerbations of chronic bronchitis in adults due to *H. influenzae* or *S. pneumoniae.*

**ACTION/KINETICS:** Sulfamethoxazole inhibits bacterial synthesis of dihydrofolic acid by competing with para-aminobenzoic acid. Trimethoprim blocks the production of tetrahydrofolic acid by inhibiting the enzyme dihydrofolate reductase. Thus, this combination blocks two consecutive steps in the bacterial biosynthesis of essential nucleic acids and proteins. The combination is rapidly and completely absorbed after PO use. **Peak plasma levels, after PO:** 1–4 hr; **after IV:** 1–1.5 hr. Urine concentrations are considerably higher than serum levels. **Sulfamethoxazole, t½, after PO:** 10–12 hr; after IV: 11.3 hr. **Trimethoprim, t½, after PO:** 8–11 hr; **after IV:** 12.8 hr. t½'s are increased significantly in those with severely impaired renal function. Sulfamethoxazole is metabolized to inactive compounds whereas trimethoprim is metabolized only to a small extent. Both are excreted through the kidneys.

**SIDE EFFECTS:** N&V, anorexia, rash, urticaria. *HEPATIC NECROSIS, PANCREATITIS, AGRANULOCYTOSIS, APLASTIC ANEMIA, STEVENS-JOHNSON SYNDROME.*

**DOSAGE: Double-Strength Tablets; Oral Suspension; Tablets**

*UTIs, shigellosis, bronchitis, acute otitis media.*

 **Adults:** 1 double strength tablet, 2 tablets, or 4 teaspoonfuls of suspension q 12 hr for 10–14 days. (*NOTE:* For shigellosis, give adult dose for 5 days.) For clients with impaired renal function the following dosage is recommended: C_CR of 15–30 mL/min: One-half the usual regimen and for C_CR less than 15 mL/min: Use is not recommended.

*Chancroid.*

 **Adults:** 1 double strength tablet twice a day for at least 7 days (alternate therapy: 4 double strength tablets in a single dose).

*Pharyngeal gonococcal infection due to penicillinase-producing*
Neisseria gonorrhoeae.
**Adults:** 720 mg trimethoprim and 3,600 mg sulfamethoxazole once daily for 5 days.

*Prophylaxis of P. carinii pneumonia.*
**Adults:** 160 mg trimethoprim and 800 mg sulfamethoxazole q 24 hr. Do not exceed a total daily dose of 320 mg trimethoprim and 1,600 mg sulfamethoxazole.

*Treatment of P. carinii pneumonia.*
**Adults:** Total daily dose of 15–20 mg/kg trimethoprim and 100 mg/kg sulfamethoxazole divided equally and given q 6 hr for 14–21 days.

*Prophylaxis of P. carinii pneumonia in immunocompromised clients.*
**Adults:** 1 double strength tablet daily.

*Traveler's diarrhea.*
**Adults:** 1 double strength tablet q 12 hr for 5 days.

*Prostatitis, acute bacterial.*
**Adults:** 1 double strength tablet twice a day until client is afebrile for 48 hr; treatment may be required for up to 30 days.

*Prostatitis, chronic bacterial.*
**Adults:** 1 double strength tablet twice a day for 4–6 weeks.

## DOSAGE: IV

*UTIs, shigellosis, acute otitis media.*
**Adults:** 8–10 mg/kg/day (based on trimethoprim) in two to four divided doses q 6, 8, or 12 hr for up to 14 days for severe UTIs or 5 days for shigellosis.

*Treatment of P. carinii pneumonia.*
**Adults:** 15–20 mg/kg/day (based on trimethoprim) in 3–4 divided doses q 6–8 hr for up to 14 days.

---

**NEED TO KNOW**

1. Do not use in megaloblastic anemia due to folate deficiency.
2. Use with caution in impaired liver or kidney function and in clients with possible folate deficiency.
3. Administer IV infusion over a 60–90 min period.

4. Do not mix the IV infusion with any other drugs or solutions.
5. Complete entire prescription and do not share.
6. Report any symptoms of persistent fever, inflammation/swelling of veins/lymph glands, N&V, rash, joint pain/swelling, mental disturbances, or lack of response.
7. Consume 2.5–3 L of fluids/day to prevent crystalluria and dehydration.
8. May experience dizziness, use caution with activities that require mental alertness.
9. Avoid prolonged sun exposure; use protective clothing, sunglasses, and sunscreen if exposure necessary.

**CLASSIFICATION(S):** Drug for erectile dysfunction

**USES:** Treatment of erectile dysfunction.

**ACTION/KINETICS:** During sexual stimulation, nitric oxide is released from nerve endings and endothelial cells in the corpus cavernosum of the penis. Nitric oxide activates the enzyme guanylate cyclase causing an increased synthesis of cyclic guanosine monophosphate (cGMP) in the smooth muscle cells of the corpus cavernosum. The cGMP in turn causes smooth muscle relaxation, allowing increased blood flow to the penis, resulting in erection. Tissue levels of cGMP are regulated by both the rate of synthesis and degradation via phosphodiesterases (PDEs). The most abundant PDE in the human corpus cavernosum is the cGMP-specific phosphodiesterase type 5 (PDE5). Thus, inhibition of PDE5 enhances erectile function by increasing the amount of cGMP. Vardenafil is a selective inhibitor of PDE5. Rapidly absorbed. **Maximum plasma levels:** 30–120 min after a single 20 mg dose. Food decreases $C_{max}$ by 18–50%. **Onset:** About 20 min; **maximum effect:** 45–90 min. **Duration:** Less than 5 hr. Eliminated primarily by hepatic metabolism by CYP3A4 and to a minor extent by CYP2C isoforms. The major metabolite, M1, is active. $t\frac{1}{2}$, **terminal:** 4–5 hr for both vardenafil and the M1 metabolite. Excreted mainly in the feces (91–95%) with a small amount in the urine (2–6%).

**SIDE EFFECTS:** Headache, dizziness, dyspepsia, nausea, diarrhea, rhinitis, sinusitis, accidental injury, back pain, flu syndrome, flushing, myalgia, rash, abnormal vision. *MI, ANGINA PECTORIS, MYOCARDIAL ISCHEMIA, ANAPHYLAXIS (INCLUDING LARYNGEAL EDEMA).*

---

**DOSAGE: Tablets**

*Erectile dysfunction.*

**Adults, initial:** 10 mg about 60 min before sexual activity. Dose may be increased to 20 mg or decreased to 5 mg based on efficacy and side effects. Maximum recommended dosing is once a day. An initial dose of 5 mg should be considered in clients 65 years and older and in those with moderate hepatic impairment.

## NEED TO KNOW

1. Do not use with regular or intermittent nitrates (due to potentiation of hypotensive effects of nitrates) or with alpha-adrenergic blockers.
2. Do not use in clients with congenital QT prolongation and those taking Class 1A (quinidine, procainamide) or Class III (amiodarone, sotalol) antiarrhythmic drugs.
3. Do not use in clients with unstable angina, hypotension, uncontrolled hypertension, recent history of stroke, life-threatening arrhythmia, MI (within the last 6 months), severe cardiac failure, severe hepatic impairment (Child-Pugh score from 10 to 15), end stage renal disease requiring dialysis, or known hereditary degenerative retinal disorders (including retinitis pigmentosa).
4. Use with caution in clients with bleeding disorders or active peptic ulceration, in those with anatomical deformation (e.g., angulation, cavernosal fibrosis, Peyronie's disease) of the penis, or in those who have conditions that may predispose them to priapism (e.g., sickle cell anemia, multiple myeloma, leukemia).
5. The initial dose in those with moderate hepatic impairment (Child-Pugh score from 7 to 9) is 5 mg; the maximum dose in those with moderate hepatic impairment should not exceed 10 mg.
6. A single dose of 2.5 mg should not be exceeded in clients taking indinavir or ritonavir. No more than a single 2.5 mg dose should be taken in a 72-hr period in those taking ritonavir.
7. A dose of 2.5 mg daily should not be exceeded in those taking ketoconazole, 400 mg/day, or itraconazole, 400 mg/day. A dose of 5 mg daily should not be exceeded in those taking ketoconazole, 200 mg/day, or itraconazole, 200 mg/day.

8. Can be taken with or without food.
9. May experience headache, flushing, upset stomach, stuffy nose, dizziness (from drop in BP), drowsiness, or abnormal vision (especially blue/green color discrimination); report any unusual, persistent, or bothersome effects.
10. Do not use any other agent for erections with this therapy.
11. Do not use more than once a day. Erections lasting more than 4 hr or painful erections lasting more than 6 hr require immediate care; penile damage may result.

---

## Varenicline tartrate      C
(var-**EN**-ih-kline)
**Rx:** Chantix.

**CLASSIFICATION(S):** Smoking deterrent
**USES:** Aid to smoking cessation treatment.
**ACTION/KINETICS:** Varenicline binds with high affinity and selectivity at α4β2 neuronal nicotinic acetylcholine receptors. The effectiveness in smoking cessation is thought to be due to the drug preventing nicotine from binding to α4β2 receptors. Thus, nicotine cannot stimulate the central nervous mesolimbic dopamine system, believed to be the neuronal mechanism underlying reinforcement and reward experienced by smoking. **Maximum plasma levels:** 3–4 hr. **Steady state levels:** 4 days. **t½, elimination:** 24 hr. Undergoes minimal metabolism with 92% excreted unchanged in the urine.
**SIDE EFFECTS:** N&V, sleep disturbances, constipation, flatulence, headache, insomnia, abnormal dreams, dysgeusia, upper respiratory tract disorder, hypertension, hyperhidrosis. *SUICIDAL IDEATION, SUICIDE, GI HEMORRHAGE, ACUTE PANCREATITIS, MI, THROMBOSIS.*

**DOSAGE: Tablets**
*Aid to smoking cessation.*
    **Adults: Dosage titration, Days 1–3:** 0.5 mg once a day; **days 4–7:** 0.5 mg twice a day. **Day 8 through end of treatment:** 1

mg twice a day. Treat clients for 12 weeks. For those who have successfully stopped smoking at the end of 12 weeks, an additional course of 12 weeks is recommended to increase further the likelihood of long-term abstinence.

## NEED TO KNOW

1. Due to decreased renal function in the elderly, use care in dose selection; consider monitoring renal function.
2. Clients who do not stop smoking during 12 weeks of initial therapy, or who relapse after treatment, should be encouraged to make another attempt after identifying and addressing the factors that contributed to the failed attempt.
3. For clients with severe impaired renal function, the recommended initial dose is 0.5 mg once a day. Then titrate as needed to a maximum of 0.5 mg twice a day. For those with end-stage renal disease undergoing hemodialysis, a maximum dosage of 0.5 mg once a day may be given if well tolerated.
4. Take after eating and with a full glass of water (8 oz/240 mL).
5. May cause drowsiness or dizziness; may be worse with alcohol or certain medicines. Do not drive or perform activities that require mental alertness until drug effects realized.
6. Do not stop drug suddenly; may cause increased irritability or difficulty sleeping.
7. May experience nausea and insomnia; report if persistent as a dose reduction may be considered.

---

## Venlafaxine hydrochloride
(ven-lah-**FAX**-een)
**Rx:** Effexor, Effexor XR.

■ **C**

**CLASSIFICATION(S):** Antidepressant, miscellaneous
**USES:** (1) Major depressive disorder. (2) Treatment of generalized anxiety disorder. (3) Treatment of social anxiety disorder (social

phobia), use extended-release product. (4) Adults with panic disorder.

**ACTION/KINETICS:** A potent inhibitor of the uptake of neuronal serotonin and norepinephrine in the CNS and a weak inhibitor of the uptake of dopamine. Has no anticholinergic, sedative, or orthostatic hypotensive effects. Well absorbed (92%); absolute bioavailability is about 45%. Metabolized in the liver by CYP2D6 and CYP3A4. The major metabolite—O-desmethylvenlafaxine (ODV)—is active. The drug and metabolite are eliminated through the kidneys. $t\frac{1}{2}$, **venlafaxine:** 5 hr; $t\frac{1}{2}$, **ODV:** 11 hr. **Time to reach steady state:** 3–4 days. The half-life of the drug and metabolite are increased in clients with impaired liver or renal function.

**SIDE EFFECTS:** Nausea, headache, somnolence, dizziness, insomnia, nervousness, constipation, asthenia, dry mouth, abnormal ejaculation/orgasm, sweating. *SEIZURES, SUICIDE ATTEMPTS, RECTAL HEMORRHAGE, UTERINE HEMORRHAGE, VAGINAL HEMORRHAGE.*

---

**DOSAGE: Tablets, Immediate-Release**

*Major depressive disorder.*

> **Adults, initial:** 75 mg/day given in two or three divided doses. Depending on the response, the dose can be increased to 150–225 mg/day in divided doses. Make dosage increments up to 75 mg/day at intervals of 4 or more days. Severely depressed clients may require 375 mg/day in divided doses.
> **Maintenance:** Periodically assess client to determine the need for maintenance treatment and the appropriate dose.

**DOSAGE: Capsules, Extended-Release**

*Major depressive disorder.*

> **Adults, initial:** 75 mg as a single dose once daily in the morning or evening at about the same time each day. For some clients it may be desirable to start at 37.5 mg/day for 4–7 days to allow adjustment to the drug before increasing to 75 mg/day. Dose can be increased by up to 75 mg no more often than every 4 days, to a maximum of 225 mg/day.

*Generalized/social anxiety disorder.*

> **Adults, initial, usual:** 75 mg/day as a single dose; if neces-

sary, the dose may be increased to 225 mg/day. Increase in increments of up to 75 mg/day at intervals of not less than 4 days. To avoid overstimulation, some may need to start with 37.5 mg/day. Take on a daily basis not on an as-needed basis. **Maintenance:** Periodically reassess the need for continuing the medication.

*Hot flushes in otherwise healthy postmenopausal women.*
**Adults:** 75 mg/day.

## NEED TO KNOW

1. Do not use with a MAOI or within 14 days of discontinuation of a MAOI.
2. Use with caution with impaired hepatic (e.g., cirrhosis) or renal (GFR = 10–70 mL/min) function, in clients with a history of mania, and in those with diseases or conditions that could affect the hemodynamic responses or metabolism.
3. Although it is possible for a geriatric client to be more sensitive, dosage adjustment is not necessary.
4. Clinical worsening and suicide risk is possible in adult clients with major depressive disorder.
5. Take with food.
6. When discontinuing after 1 week or more of therapy, taper dose to minimize risk of withdrawal syndrome. If drug has been taken for 6 weeks or more, taper dose gradually over a 2-week period.
7. Abrupt discontinuation or dose reduction of venlafaxine (at various doses) may be associated with the appearance of new symptoms (frequency increased with increased dose level and with longer duration of treatment). Symptoms include agitation, anorexia, anxiety, confusion, impaired coordination, diarrhea, dizziness, dry mouth, dysphoric mood, fasciculation, fatigue, headaches, hypomania, insomnia, nausea, nervousness, nightmares, sensory disturbances (including shock-like electrical sensations), somnolence, sweating, tremor, vertigo, and vomiting.

and promptly consumed without chewing and followed with a glass of water to ensure complete swallowing of the pellets. Drug may impair appetite and induce weight loss; report if excessive.

9. Report any rash, hives, or other allergic manifestations immediately. May experience anxiety, palpitations, headaches, and constipation; report if persistent or intolerable.

10. Due to the possibility of suicide, high-risk clients should be observed closely during initial therapy. Prescriptions should be written for the smallest quantity to reduce the risk of overdose.

## Warfarin sodium      X
(WAR-far-in)
**Rx:** Coumadin, Jantoven.

**CLASSIFICATION(S):** Anticoagulant, coumarin derivative
**USES:** (1) Prophylaxis and treatment of venous thrombosis and its extension. (2) Prophylaxis and treatment of atrial fibrillation with embolization. (3) Prophylaxis and treatment of pulmonary embolism. (4) Prophylaxis and treatment of thromboembolic complications associated with atrial fibrillation.
**ACTION/KINETICS:** Interferes with synthesis of vitamin K–dependent clotting factors resulting in depletion of clotting factors II, VII, IX, and X. Has no direct effect on an established thrombus although therapy may prevent further extension of a formed clot as well as secondary thromboembolic problems. Well absorbed from the GI tract although food affects the rate (but not the extent) of absorption. Suitable for parenteral administration. **Peak activity:** 1.5–3 days; **duration:** 2–5 days. **t½:** 1–2.5 days. Metabolized in the liver and inactive metabolites are excreted through the urine and feces.
**SIDE EFFECTS:** Bleeding/hemorrhage.

**DOSAGE: IV; Tablets**

*Induction.*

**Adults, initial:** 5–10 mg/day for 2–4 days; **then,** adjust dose based on prothrombin or international normalized ratio (INR) determinations. A lower dose should be used in geriatric or debilitated clients or clients with increased sensitivity.

*Maintenance.*

**Adults:** 2–10 mg/day, based on prothrombin or INR.

*Prevent blood clots with prosthetic heart valve replacement.*

**Adults:** 2–5 mg daily.

**NEED TO KNOW**

1. Use of a large loading dose (30 mg) is not recommended due to increased risk of hemorrhage and lack of more rapid protection.
2. Geriatric clients are at an increased risk for bleeding, thromboembolic events, and atrial fibrillation.
3. Anticoagulant use in the following clients leads to increased risk: Trauma, infection, renal insufficiency, sprue, vitamin K deficiency, severe to moderate hypertension, polycythemia vera, severe allergic disorders, vasculitis, indwelling catheters, severe diabetes, anaphylactic disorders, surgery or trauma resulting in large exposed raw surfaces.
4. Warfarin is responsible for more adverse drug interactions than any other group. Clients on anticoagulant therapy must be monitored carefully each time a drug is added or withdrawn.
5. Frequent monitoring of PT/INR is recommended during the first week of therapy, during adjustment periods, and monthly thereafter.
6. To transfer from heparin therapy, give heparin and warfarin together from the first day (delayed onset of oral anticoagulant effects). Alternatively, warfarin may be started on the third to sixth day of heparin therapy.

7. Take oral warfarin as prescribed and at the same time each day; must be compliant with therapy. Do not change brands of drug; may alter response. Avoid eating large amounts of grapefruit or drinking grapefruit or cranberry juice.

8. Avoid IM shots, activities/contact sports that may cause injury or cuts and bruises. Use a soft toothbrush, electric razor to shave, wear shoes and use a night light to avoid falls at night.

9. Report immediately unusual bruising/bleeding, dark brown or blood-tinged body secretions, injury or trauma, dizziness, abdominal pain or swelling, back pain, severe headaches, and joint swelling and pain.

10. Avoid OTC drugs. Check prior to taking any OTC drugs that have anticoagulant-type effects such as salicylates, NSAIDs, steroids, vitamin K, mineral preparations from health food stores, vitamins, herbal teas, herbals, alcohol. Check with provider to see whether to continue baby aspirin. Should be done with acute myocardial infarction to prevent recurrence.

11. Wear identification and alert all providers of anticoagulant therapy.

12. Unusual hair loss and itching are common with the elderly; advise to report if intolerable or skin breakdown occurs.

13. Elderly are more prone to developing bleeding complications. Many elderly use multiple pharmacies and shop for value; stress need to know what they are taking and why and to carry the name and dosage of ALL drugs prescribed. Remind not to skip a dose as drug works for only 24 hr and must be read-ministered in order to be effective. Carry list of all meds/vitamins/herbals prescribed/consumed to all visits to provider/pharmacy.

## Zolpidem tartrate
(ZOL-pih-dem)

(Immediate-Release) **B**
(Extended-Release) **C**

**Rx:** Ambien, Ambien CR, Tovalt ODT, **C-IV.**

**CLASSIFICATION(S):** Sedative-hypnotic, nonbenzodiazepine

**USES: Immediate-Release Tablets:** Short-term treatment of insomnia (7–10 days of use). Re-evaluate if hypnotics are to be taken for more than 2–3 weeks. **Extended-Release/Orally Disintegrating Tablets:** Treatment of insomnia characterized by difficulties with sleep onset and/or sleep maintenance.

**ACTION/KINETICS:** May act by subunit modulation of the GABA receptor chloride channel macromolecular complex resulting in sedative, anticonvulsant, anxiolytic, and myorelaxant properties. Specifically, it binds to the omega-1 receptor preferentially. No evidence of residual next-day effects or rebound insomnia at usual doses; little evidence for memory impairment. Sleep time spent in stage 3 to 4 (deep sleep) was comparable to placebo with only inconsistent, minor changes in REM sleep at recommended doses. Rapidly absorbed from the GI tract. **t$\frac{1}{2}$, elimination, immediate-release:** About 2.5 hr (increased in geriatric clients and those with impaired hepatic function). **t$\frac{1}{2}$ elimination, orally disintegrating:** 3.5 hr (nighttime dosing). **t$\frac{1}{2}$, elimination, extended-release:** 2.8 hr. Food decreases the bioavailability of zolpidem. Metabolized in the liver; inactive metabolites are excreted primarily through the urine.

**SIDE EFFECTS: Immediate-Release/Oral Disintegrating:** Dizziness, drowsiness, drugged feeling, headache, nausea, diarrhea, dyspepsia, myalgia, URTI. **Extended-Release:** Headache, somnolence, dizziness, nausea, diarrhea, nasopharyngitis.

**DOSAGE: Tablets, Immediate-Release; Tablets, Orally Disintegrating**

*Hypnotic.*

**Adults, individualized, usual:** 10 mg just before bedtime. In the elderly or in hepatic insufficiency, use an initial dose of 5 mg.

## DOSAGE: Tablets, Extended-Release

*Hypnotic.*

**Adults:** Individualize dose. 12.5 mg just before bedtime. For elderly or debilitated clients, give 6.25 mg just before bedtime.

---

### NEED TO KNOW

1. Use with caution and at reduced dosage in clients with impaired hepatic function, in compromised respiratory function, in those with impaired renal function, and in clients with S&S of depression.
2. Impaired motor or cognitive performance after repeated use or unusual sensitivity to hypnotic drugs may be noted in geriatric or debilitated clients.
3. Limit therapy to 7–10 days. Reevaluate if the drug is required for more than 2–3 weeks.
4. Do not exceed 10 mg daily of the immediate-release or oral disintegrating tablets or 12.5 mg of the extended-release tablets.
5. Take only as directed, whole, on an empty stomach with a full glass of water just before going to bed. For faster sleep onset, do not administer with or immediately after a meal.
6. If using orally disintegrating tablets, open the blister pack and peel back the foil on the blister. Do not push the tablet through the foil. Remove the tablet and place it in the mouth where it will dissolve in seconds; then swallow with saliva. Can be taken with or without water. Do not chew, break, or split the tablet. Do not give with or immediately after a meal.
7. Avoid alcohol, caffeine, chocolate after 4 p.m., and any unprescribed or OTC drugs.
8. Do not perform any activity that requires mental or physical alertness until drug effects realized.

## Calculating Body Surface Area and Body Mass Index

### Body Surface Area (BSA) Calculator

Use the following formulas to calculate the body surface area (BSA) for drug administration. These formulas replace the BSA Nomogram.

BSA (metric) = $\sqrt{(\text{ht [cm]} \times \text{wt [kg]})/3600}$

BSA (English) = $\sqrt{(\text{ht [in]} \times \text{wt [lb]})/3131}$

### Body Mass Index (BMI) Calculator

You may calculate your BMI to assess if you are overweight

1. Multiply your weight in pounds by 703
2. Multiply your height in inches times itself
3. Divide the first number by the second to give your BMI

For example:

You weigh 190 lb and are 5'5" (65") tall

1. 190 x 703 = 133,579
2. 65 x 65 = 4,225
3. 133,579 divided by 4,225 = 31.6

Your BMI is 31.6

A BMI under 18.5 indicates that you are underweight

A BMI between 18.5 and 24.9 is considered a healthy weight

If the BMI is between 25 and 29.9 you are moderately overweight

If the BMI is 30 or more you are extremely obese

A precalculated BMI chart is available in most provider offices.

A precalculated BMI chart is available from the National Institutes of Health at:

http://www.nhlbi.nih.gov/guidelines/obesity/bmi_tbl.htm

# APPENDIX 2

## Elements of a Prescription

To safely communicate the exact elements desired on a prescription, the following items should be addressed:

A. **The prescriber:** Name, address, phone number, and associated practice/specialty.

B. **The client:** Name, age/birthdate, address, and any allergies of record.

C. **The prescription itself:** Name of the medication (generic or trade); dosage form and quantity to be dispensed (e.g., number of tablets or capsules, 1 vial, 1 tube, volume of liquid); the strength of the medication (e.g., 125-mg tablets, 250 mg/5 mL, 80 mg/1 mL, 10%); and directions for use (e.g., 1 tablet PO 3 times per day; 2 gtt to each eye 4 times per day; 1 teaspoonful PO q 8 hr for 10 days; apply a thin film to lesions twice a day for 14 days).

D. **Other elements:** Date prescription is written, signature of the provider, number of refills, provider number: state license number and Drug Enforcement Agency (DEA) number (when applicable), and brand-product-only indication (when applicable).

A typical prescription follows:

A. Julia Bryan, MSN, RN, CPNP
Pediatric Associates
1611 Kirkwood Highway
Wilmington, DE 19805
302-645-8261

Date: July 10, 20XX

B. For: Kathryn Woods, Age 8

Rx Amoxicillin susp. 250 mg/5 mL
Disp. 150 mL
Sig: 1 teaspoon PO q 8 hr x 10 days

Refills: 0 Provider signature
Provider/State license number

**Interpretation of prescription:** The above prescription is written by Certified Pediatric Nurse Practitioner Julia Bryan for Kathryn Woods and is for amoxicillin suspension. The concentration desired is 250 mg/5 mL. The directions for taking the medication are 1 teaspoon (i.e., 5 mL) by mouth every 8 hr for 10 days. The prescriber wants 150 mL dispensed and no refills are allowed.

## Drug/Food Interactions

### A. DRUGS THAT SHOULD BE TAKEN WHILE FASTING

Alendronate

Digoxin (avoid high fiber cereals and oatmeal)

Lansoprazole

Levodopa (not with high protein foods; meals delay absorption and peak plasma concentration; avoid caffeine)

Trimethoprim

### B. DRUGS THAT SHOULD BE TAKEN WITH FOOD

Allopurinol (after meal)

Diclofenac

Glyburide

Lovastatin

Metoprolol

Naproxen

Propranolol

### C. CONSTIPATING AGENTS

Antacids

Anticholinergic drugs

Anticonvulsants

Antihistamines

Antiparkinsonian drugs

BP meds (calcium channel blockers)

Clonidine

Corticosteroids

Diuretics

Ganglionic blocking agents

Iron supplements

Laxatives (when abused)

Lithium

MAO Inhibitors

Muscle relaxants

NSAIDs

Octreotide

Opioids

Phenothiazines

Prostaglandin synthesis inhibitors

Tranquilizers

Tricyclic antidepressants

## D. DIARRHEAL AGENTS

Adrenergic neuron blockers: reserpine, guanethidine

Antacids (Mg containing) $H_2$ receptor antagonists (i.e., ranitidine) PPIs (i.e., omeprazole)

Antiarrhythmics (i.e., quinidine)

Antibiotics (especially broad spectrum agents)

Antihypertensives (beta blockers, ACE Inhibitors)

Anti-inflammatory drugs (NSAIDs, colchicine)

Chemotherapy agents

Cholinergic agonists and cholinesterase inhibitors

Glucophage

Metoclopramide

Misoprostol

Osmotic and stimulant laxatives

Theophylline

## E. TYRAMINE CONTAINING FOODS

*Moderate amounts of tyramine:*

Banana peel

Broad beans

Cheese (all except cream cheese and cottage cheese)

Chianti, vermouth

Concentrated yeast extracts/Brewer's yeast

Fermented cabbage products: sauerkraut, kimchee

Fermented soy products: fermented bean curd, soya bean paste, miso soup

Hydrolyzed protein extracts for sauces, soups, gravies

Imitation cheese

Liquid and powdered protein supplements

Meat extracts

Nonalcoholic beers

Prepared meats (sausage, chopped liver, pate, salami, mortadella)
Raspberries
Some non-United States brands of beer
Yeast products

*Significant amounts of tyramine:*
Avocado
Chocolate
Cream from fresh pasteurized milk
Distilled spirits
Peanuts
Red and white wines, port wines
Soy sauce
Yogurt

## F. FOODS CONTAINING GOITROGENS

Asparagus
Broccoli
Brussels sprouts
Cabbage
Cauliflower
Kale
Lettuce
Millet
Mustard
Other leafy green vegetables
Peaches
Peanuts
Peas
Radishes
Rutabaga
Soy beans
Spinach
Strawberries
Turnip greens
Watercress

## G. COUMARIN ANTICOAGULANTS AND DIETARY EFFECTS

Consumption of vitamin K-enriched foods may counteract the effects of anticoagulants since the drugs act through antagonism of vitamin K. Advise client on anticoagulants to maintain a steady, consistent intake of vitamin K-containing foods. The drug monograph for warfarin clearly lists these foods. Additionally, certain herbal teas (green tea, buckeye, horse chestnut, Woodruff, tonka beans, melitot) contain natural coumarins that can potentiate the effects of coumadin and should be avoided. Large amounts of avocado also potentiate the drug's effects. Brussels sprouts, broccoli, spinach, kale, turnip greens, and other cruciferous vegetables increase the catabolism of warfarin thereby decreasing its anticoagulant activities. Caffeinated beverages (i.e., cola, coffee, tea, hot chocolate, chocolate milk) can affect therapy. Alcohol intake of more than three drinks per day can affect clotting times. Herbal supplements can also affect bleeding time: Coenzyme Q10 is structurally similar to vitamin K, feverfew, garlic, and ginseng. Avoid herbal medications while on warfarin therapy.

## H. GENERAL DRUG CLASS RECOMMENDATIONS

**ACE inhibitors**: Take captopril and moexipril 1 hr before or 2 hr after meals; food decreases absorption. Avoid high potassium foods as ACE increases $K^+$.

**Analgesic/Antipyretic**: Take on an empty stomach as food may slow the absorption.

**Antacids**: Take 1 hr after or between meals. Avoid dairy foods as the protein in them can increase stomach acid.

**Anti-anxiety agents**: Caffeine may cause excitability, nervousness, and hyperactivity lessening the anti-anxiety drug effects.

**Antibiotics**: Penicillin generally should be taken on an empty stomach; may take with food if GI upset occurs. Do not mix with acidic foods: coffee, citrus fruits, and tomatoes; the acid interferes with absorption of penicillin, ampicillin, erythromycin, and cloxacillin.

**Anticoagulants**: High vitamin K produces blood-clotting substance and may reduce drug effectiveness. Vitamin E greater than 400 IU may prolong clotting time and increase bleeding risk.

**Antidepressant drugs**: May be taken with or without food.

**Antifungals**: Avoid taking with dairy products; avoid alcohol.

**Antihistamines**: Take on an empty stomach to increase effectiveness.

**Bronchodilators with theophylline**: High-fat meals may increase bioavailability while high-carbohydrate meals may decrease it. Food increases absorption of Theo-24 and Uniphyl which may cause increased N&V, headache, and irritability.

**Cephalosporins**: Take on an empty stomach 1 hr before or 2 hr after meals. May take with food if GI upset occurs.

salty food and natural black licorice as these increase K and Mg losses. Large doses of vitamin D can elevate blood pressure.

**H$_2$ blockers:** May take with or without regard to food.

**HMG-CoA reductase inhibitors:** Take lovastatin with the evening meal to enhance absorption.

**Laxatives:** Avoid dairy foods as calcium can decrease absorption.

**Macrolides:** Take on an empty stomach 1 hr before or 2 hr after meals. May take with food for GI upset.

**MAO inhibitors:** Have many dietary restrictions, so follow dietary guidelines as prescribed. Foods or alcoholic beverages containing tyramine may cause a fatal increase in BP.

**Narcotic analgesics:** Avoid alcohol as it may increase sedative effects.

**Nitroimadazole (metronidazole):** Avoid alcohol or food prepared with alcohol for at least three days after finishing the medicine. Alcohol may cause nausea, abdominal cramps, vomiting, headaches, and flushing.

**NSAIDs:** Take with food or milk to prevent irritation of the stomach.

**Quinolones:** Take on an empty stomach 1 hr before or 2 hr after meals. May take with food for GI upset but avoid calcium containing foods such as milk, yogurt, vitamins/minerals containing iron, and antacids because they decrease drug concentrations. Caffeine containing products may lead to excitability and nervousness.

**Sulfonamides:** Take on an empty stomach 1 hr before or 2 hr after meals. May take with food if GI upset occurs.

**Tetracyclines:** Take on an empty stomach 1 hr before or 2 hr after meals. May take with food but avoid dairy products, antacids, and vitamins containing iron.

# APPENDIX 4

## Drugs Whose Effects Are Modified by Grapefruit Juice

Increasing numbers of drugs have been identified whose effects are modified by short-term or chronic use of grapefruit juice. This effect is likely due to furanocoumarins that are present in grapefruit juice. The following is a representative list of those drugs, including the mechanism for the altered drug effect. The most frequent result is an increase in plasma levels of the drug, which may increase the risk of side effects.

| Drug | Mechanism for Altered Effect |
| --- | --- |
| Amlodipine | ↑ Plasma amlodipine levels R/T ↓ liver metabolism |
| Atorvastatin | ↑ Plasma atorvastatin levels |
| Budesonide | ↑ Plasma budesonide levels |
| Digoxin | ↑ Plasma digoxin levels |
| Estrogens | ↑ Plasma levels of 17-beta estradiol/estrone combination |
| Fluvoxamine | ↑ Fluvoxamine mean AUC and $C_{max}$ |
| Lovastatin | ↑ Plasma lovastatin levels R/T ↓ liver metabolism |
| Sildenafil | ↑ Plasma sildenafil levels R/T ↓ liver metabolism |
| Simvastatin | ↑ Plasma simvastatin levels R/T ↓ liver metabolism |
| Triazolam | ↑ Plasma triazolam levels R/T ↓ liver metabolism |

# INDEX

**Boldface** = generic drug name

George R. Spratto, PhD

*All the information you need,
right at your fingertips!*

Quick access to essential drug information for
geriatric patients is available with the portable,
pocket-sized *Delmar's Mini Guide to Geriatric
Drugs.*

Key information for 100 drugs includes:
- Pronunciation
- Classification
- Uses
- Action/Kinetics
- Side Effects
- Dosages
- Need to Know

Also, a complementary PDA download option is
provided for even more versatility!

*Delmar's Mini Guide to Geriatric Drugs—
your partner in geriatric nursing.*

ISBN-13: 978-1-4283-2003-1
ISBN-10: 1-4283-2003-2

9 781428 320031